EVOLUTION OF THE LEARNING BRAIN

How does learning transform us biologically?

What learning processes do we share with bacteria, jellyfish and monkeys?

Is technology impacting on our evolution and what might the future hold for the learning brain?

These are just some of the questions Paul Howard-Jones explores on a fascinating journey through 3.5 billion years of brain evolution, and discovers what it all means for how we learn today.

Along the way, we discover

- how the *E. coli* in our stomachs learn to find food
- why a little nap can help bees find their way home
- the many ways that action, emotion and social interaction have shaped our ability to learn
- the central role of learning in our rise to top predator.

An accessible writing style and numerous illustrations make *Evolution of the Learning Brain* an enthralling combination of biology, neuroscience and educational insight. Howard-Jones provides a fresh perspective on the nature of human learning that is exhaustively researched, exploring the implications of our most distant past for twenty-first-century education.

Paul Howard-Jones is Professor of Neuroscience and Education at the School of Education, University of Bristol. He is a cognitive neuroscientist, educational expert and broadcaster.

EVOLUTION OF THE LEARNING BRAIN

Or How You Got To Be So Smart . . .

Paul Howard-Jones

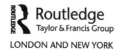

Routledge
Taylor & Francis Group

LONDON AND NEW YORK

First published 2018
by Routledge
2 Park Square, Milton Park, Abingdon, Oxon OX14 4RN

and by Routledge
711 Third Avenue, New York, NY 10017

Routledge is an imprint of the Taylor & Francis Group, an informa business

British Library Cataloguing in Publication Data
A catalogue record for this book is available from the British Library

Library of Congress Cataloging in Publication Data
Names: Howard-Jones, Paul, author.
Title: Evolution of the learning brain ; or how you got to be so smart ... /
    Paul Howard-Jones.
Other titles: How you got to be so smart ...
Description: Abingdon, Oxon ; New York, NY : Routledge, 2018. |
    Includes bibliographical references.
Identifiers: LCCN 2017031433 (print) | LCCN 2017052387 (ebook) |
    ISBN 9781138824454 (hbk) | ISBN 9781138824461 (pbk) |
    ISBN 9781315150857 (ebk)
Subjects: LCSH: Learning—Physiological aspects. | Neurosciences. |
    Cognition. | Brain—Evolution.
Classification: LCC QP408 (ebook) | LCC QP408 .H685 2018 (print) |
    DDC 612.8/233—dc23
LC record available at https://lccn.loc.gov/2017031433

ISBN: 978-1-138-82445-4 (hbk)
ISBN: 978-1-138-82446-1 (pbk)
ISBN: 978-1-315-15085-7 (ebk)

Typeset in Bembo
by Swales & Willis Ltd, Exeter, Devon, UK

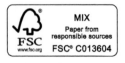

MIX
Paper from
responsible sources
FSC® C013604

Printed and bound by CPI Group (UK) Ltd, Croydon, CR0 4YY

For my dad, who would often remind us: "Give a man a fish, and you feed him for a day. Teach a man to fish, and you feed him for a lifetime."

(anon.)

CONTENTS

ACKNOWLEDGEMENTS

While I must take sole responsibility for all views, errors, over-simplifications and omissions, I would like to thank the experts who provided comment on various sections of the book and helped to greatly improve it. These are (in alphabetical order): Dr Jane Ashby (Central Michigan University), Professor Rafal Bogacz (University of Oxford), Professor Richard William Byrne (University of St Andrews), Dr Fiona Coward (Bournemouth University), Dr Kate Fenton (University of the West of England), Dr Thomas Fenton (Technical University of Denmark), Dr Régine Kolinsky (Université Libre de Bruxelles), Professor Jérôme Prado (National Center for Scientific Research), Professor Charles Snowdon (University of Wisconsin-Madison), Professor Michael Thomas (Birkbeck College, University of London) and Professor Michael Walling (Rose Bruford College).

ACKNOWLEDGEMENTS

1

THE IDEA OF EVOLUTION

THE ODDEST THING IS that you're not quite the same person as you were a few seconds ago. You have a memory of picking up this book, and this memory has joined others held somewhere in your biology: how you came to be here today, who you are and even how to read these words.

Something must change amongst the atoms and molecules of your body for you to learn and remember these things. Learning, in other words, is transformative in a very concrete sense – it changes not just our mental world but also our biological form. Learning often accumulates so gradually and quietly that the changes go unnoticed. But some ideas are so profound they entirely alter a person's view of themselves and what's around them. And when that idea spreads, it can transform others until the world itself seems changed.

On 15 September 1834, the seeds of one such idea were waiting to be discovered – perhaps the biggest scientific idea of all. The theory of evolution would help us understand how the diverse abilities of species came about, including our transformative ability to learn. On this day, by a small volcanic island 200 miles off the coast of Ecuador, a rowing boat was launched from the HMS Beagle. Its occupants negotiated it along a treacherous and abrasive coastline. Eventually, the crew found a patch of black sand where their craft could avoid being scuppered. A young Charles Darwin stepped out onto San Cristobal Island, one of the *Encantada*, or enchanted isles (aka "The Galapagos"). These islands had been a foggy sanctuary for pirates raiding Spanish galleons and Darwin was also a treasure seeker – of a type. He was hunting specimens of local animals, but this island did not look promising. In his diary he wrote: "Nothing could be less inviting than the first appearance". He didn't know it then, but the treasures he was about to discover would play a critical role in solving the "mystery of mysteries": how life evolves, and how one species can become another.

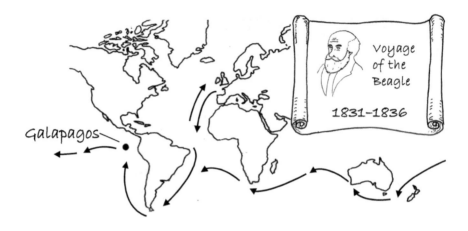

The observations and specimens that Darwin amassed would help him launch the most influential and important theory of our time. And yet, Darwin was not a qualified scientist. Like many young men of his age, he had been pursuing leisure interests while postponing a "proper job", and he was especially fond of collecting beetles and bugs. He had dropped out of medical school and been pushed into clerical training in Cambridge in readiness for the Church – then the last resort for hopeless young men from good homes. His suitability for the Church was tainted by a dwindling faith and little interest in his studies but the consolation would be a rural parish with the time and opportunity to pursue his collecting. Fate, however, had something else in store. Cambridge led to regular contact and then friendship with a Botany professor called Henslow, with whom Darwin enjoyed many long rambles and collecting expeditions in the surrounding countryside. When Henslow turned down a trip on a survey ship called the Beagle, he suggested Darwin should go. Its captain, Fitzroy, mindful of his predecessor becoming severely depressed and shooting himself, was keen to find company for the two-year voyage ahead. The captain needed someone to eat with, someone who could engage in interesting conversation and keep his demons in check. A naturalist with the skills to collect some interesting specimens would, of course, be a bonus.

In 1836, after five years, Darwin arrived back from his voyage ecstatic to be once more at his father's home and amongst his sisters. Never again need he feel the seasickness that had followed him around the world. Within days, however, the family welcome had given way to a whirl of social and scientific engagements. His letters from abroad, giving reports of strange animals, breath-taking geology and fascinating peoples, had whetted the appetites of the intellectual and chattering classes. News of his return was spreading. His celebrity status meant dinner invitations, and the opportunity to regale and entice possible funders with his South American tales. While society events rarely excited Darwin, he knew that networking would be vital for establishing himself as a scientist. He would need help from those with scientific credentials, and he would need money, to ensure he could catalogue, research and exhibit his specimens. Between the dinners he toured the institutions where he might be allowed to unpack and place parts of his collection: the Linnaean and British Museum, and the scientific societies. At the Zoological Society, he presented 80 mammals and 450 birds, on the condition that they were mounted properly and described. Amongst these were the famous Darwin finches, although at the time Darwin thought they probably all fed together as the same species, and had no sense they had adapted to different environmental niches. At the Society, the "Superintendent" John Gould quickly perceived he was in possession of a new group of finches containing 12 different species. The media was contacted and Darwin's birds were set out for display. Within a few weeks, the discovery was paraded by the President of the Geological Society at a meeting where Darwin was elected onto its council. Darwin had been slow to understand he was collecting new species but, in fairness, what counts as a new species remains a subject of debate even today (see box overleaf). Now, however, this realisation stirred an all-important question in him: why is present and past life on any one spot so closely related?

Within 18 months, Darwin was married, financially independent and living off Gower Street in the centre of London. The massive task of cataloguing, describing and publishing his specimens had really only just begun, and here he was ideally placed close to the institutions and societies that could, if he kept them sweet, support his work. But he was already pondering other, more dangerous issues, ones he had to keep from his new scientific friends for fear of alienating them. Darwin's analysis of life's diversity on the Galapagos and its island-specific variation was confronting him with more inescapable questions, such as "Why, on these tiny islands so recently emerged from the sea, were so many beings created slightly different from their South American counterparts?" In 1837, he opened a secret notebook (the "B" notebook) and began to write his thoughts on transmutation – the changing of one species into another. According to his theory, new species were constantly being generated by evolution, rather than appearing randomly or via divine design. Darwin based his arguments on three observable

Speciation and extinction

The concept of a species is a fuzzy one. When can we say there's enough difference between two evolving populations to claim we have two species? One widely used definition claims "speciation" has occurred when the two groups can no longer breed with each other.[1] Most commonly this happens when a significant number of the population becomes physically isolated due to migration or, as may have happened in the Galapagos, their habitat becomes fragmented. Within this smaller sample, inbreeding can result in a much faster rate of inherited change.

Since Darwin collected his finds on the Galapagos, small island-specific changes in its birds have been seen over just a few decades, as their environment has changed. Those birds who, simply due to random mutation, had beaks slightly more suited to the environment became naturally selected as a result.[2] Over a longer time, these changes can accumulate, explaining how different finch species have evolved and come to inhabit different islands, each adapted to the food supply offered by their island. For example, in these finches that were categorised by Gould, the beaks of 1 and 2 (opposite) are ideal for crushing large, hard seeds. While 3 has a beak ideal for grasping larger insects on the ground, 4, unlike these other finches, has the ability to catch and feed on flying insects.

When you think of the natural variation within humans, it doesn't seem so surprising that Darwin initially thought his finches were the same species. In addition to the normal variation within a species, another challenge of spotting species is that the "can only breed with each other" definition cannot apply to all life forms. It cannot, for example, apply to prokaryotes (single-celled organisms without a nucleus) since these do not reproduce sexually. These represent half the Earth's biomass and the great majority of its "species".

facts: 1) more offspring are produced than can survive; 2) trait differences between individuals influence their ability to survive and reproduce; and 3) these trait differences are heritable. On this basis, the argument follows that trait differences favouring greater fitness are more likely to be passed on, i.e. organisms evolve by a process of natural selection (see box on pp. 6–7).

But it would be another two decades before this idea was published. Why the delay? After all, you could argue the idea wasn't *that* new. In ancient Greece, philosophers had already disputed how easily and fluidly such transmutation might occur. Aristotle had suggested all living forms were variations on a defined set of fixed possibilities or "ideas". By the eighteenth century, notions of a fixed cosmic order had mostly vanished from scientific thinking about the physical world, but the living world was closer to

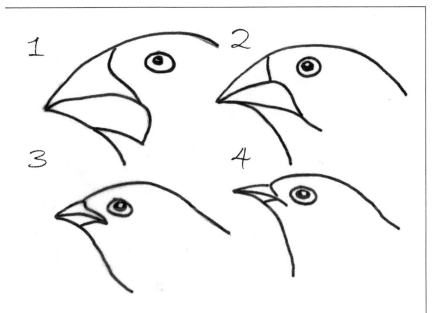

Compared with its beginning, defining the end of a species is much more straightforward. Almost all species known to have shared our planet are now extinct and it seems fair to assume that extinction is the fate of every species. Extinction occurs continuously but spikes have occurred in the background rate. The most dramatic on record was the Permian-Triassic extinction (252 Myr) when 96% of species disappeared. We are presently living (for the time being at least) through the Holocene extinction with rates 100–1000 times greater than background levels, with our own species implicated as the primary cause and global warming set to increase rates further.

the divine. Biology in Darwin's day still clung to notions of fixed natural types, created as part of some supernatural plan. This dominant notion of intelligent design had resisted suggestions by thinkers such as Lamarck that species might transmute. These "free-thinkers" included Darwin's grandfather Erasmus who, as a man of the Enlightenment, was contemptuous of the idea that God, rather than Nature, created the species. Erasmus was a renowned physician, lover of liberty, supporter of women's education and staunch opponent of slavery. But his family found many of his views concerning, since his unorthodoxy had gone further. Erasmus enjoyed writing erotic verse and prescribed sex for hypochondria, while his beliefs about evolution proposed "the strongest and most active animal should propagate the species, which should thence become improved". (That may explain

Natural selection

Though evolution tends to be slow and gradual, dramatic changes in the environment can bring about change more rapidly. The most famously observed example of Natural Selection is the pepper moth. Before 1811, only light-coloured pepper moths were known in the UK.

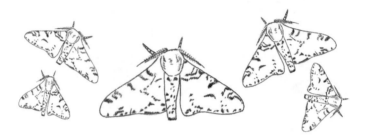

However, by 1848, at the end of the Industrial Revolution, a drastic increase in the dark-coloured variety was recorded around the industrial city of Manchester, where trees were often covered with soot. The Clean Air Act in the 1950s was followed by a decline in the number of dark relative to lighter-coloured pepper moths.[3]

why, in addition to the dozen children with his wives, he also had two with his children's governess.) In Darwin's family, evolutionary thinking was already associated with irreligious and immoral thoughts and behaviour – all threats to the status quo of respectable society. While Darwin remained uninterested in religion, his wife was devout in her faith and anxious about his ideas. Her anxiety worried him greatly.

Darwin knew that the damage potential for grand ideas about the origin of species extended well beyond his family. He was aware that evolutionary ideas can be exploited by both left- and right-wing politicians, much as they continue to be today. Since returning home, the gathering tumult in England was providing a lesson in the dangers. The Rev. Thomas Malthus had suggested that any population size, if unchecked, would grow exponentially and outpace the food supply. Darwin had made a similar observation in the natural world, i.e. that more offspring are produced than can normally survive. Malthus, however, made his own interpretation of this for policy – and had begun reflecting on what options should be implemented for checking population growth. He proposed not only that moral

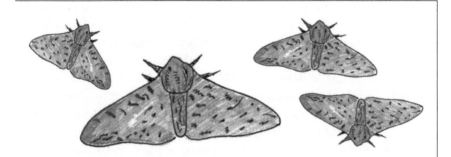

Evolutionary theory prompted the idea that a light colour was more effective camouflage for these moths in a clean environment and a dark colour was a better way to survive predators when the environment became polluted.[4,5] Those moths whose colour was better fitted to their background survived and reproduced in greater numbers, and so that colour became predominant in the population. Understanding pepper moths from an evolutionary perspective helps us appreciate, understand and explore how they are "fitted" to their environment. It prompted further experiments that have confirmed the importance of colour for an individual moth's survival[6] and further questions about the genetics of moth colour.

restraints should be encouraged (e.g. sexual abstinence), but also that those suffering poverty and other circumstances he regarded as "defects" should not be allowed to reproduce. He promoted these policies as the available options to disease, starvation and war. On this basis, the poor did not need charity since this might expand their numbers; instead, they just needed control and discipline. Buoyed by Malthusian principles, the "New Poor Law" meant no more outdoor charity. Either the poor competed with everyone else or they would find themselves in the new workhouses that were springing up everywhere. Those outraged by inequities such as this "punishment of the poor" came together in a nation-wide protest movement (the Chartists) to support a people's charter. Riots ensued, soldiers were called out and some demonstrators were shot. One incident hemmed the Darwin family into their London home as troops charged crowds a few yards from their door.

A few days after those troop charges, in 1842, Darwin, along with his wife and children, retreated to a new and somewhat desolate home in the Kentish North Downs – far away from the chaos, unrest and noise of a restless London. This would be where Darwin could study and develop his theory in the solitude he now loved. Gone were the sounds of the Chartist riots in the streets below, but the thought of "coming out" with his ideas was still not attractive. He was no longer the naïve young man who had boarded the Beagle to pursue his hobby and avoid a job in the Church. If not picked up by Malthusians, his ideas might be adored by revolutionaries seeking to destroy the Church's power and disrupt the class structure his family benefited from. The Church's doctrine of God-given difference was key to its authority. It justified why some might be poor and powerless and others were rich and ruling. This underpinned the religious case for keeping things broadly as they were, protecting the wealthy Church and the elite that supported it. In contrast – Darwin's theory suggested all living creatures shared the same first ancestor – that we were all part of the same web of life. It dispensed with the notion of a divine decree that separated the human from the non-human, or indeed any type of human from any other. This sense of unity and its consequent equality would be a gift to those wanting to challenge the current order, and who were now taunting the Church as a "harlot" in bed with the state. The ideas spawning in Darwin's mind were contrary to his life as a pastor's son, his yearning for a quiet country life, the strong religious sentiments of his wife and the sentiments of his own social class.

The inner conflict all this created has been linked to the many illnesses that marred Darwin's life, and blamed for the incredible delay of 20 years in publishing his theory. Yet publish he did, finally prompted into a sense of urgency when Alfred Wallace sent him an essay proposing a very similar idea. There was now no point in holding back because Wallace would publish anyway. It is fortunate for all of us that Darwin stepped into the ring at this point to promote his theory with Wallace. The ensuing debate would need his unique skills and his massive body of evidence to ensure it was taken seriously and appropriately interpreted. His scientific rigour and humanism would help illuminate evolution as a concept that unified all humanity, and all life. After his long period of covert self-examination and agonising, he finally set the date for publicly committing himself. The event was to be a joint publication with Wallace, presented at the Linnean Society in Piccadilly.

In the end, the meeting itself was something of a non-event. Darwin had recently lost his youngest child to scarlet fever and stayed at home grief-stricken; Wallace was abroad. It was the final meeting before summer recess and a small audience of about 30 members listened without comment as the secretary of the society read out the paper. The President walked out of the meeting, lamenting how the year had been disappointing, with no "striking discoveries which at once revolutionize, so to speak, [our] department of science".

Ironically, perhaps, the lack of clamour had an encouraging effect on Darwin. He had now shown his colours and, despite all the anxiety, no-one seemed very bothered. About a year later, he published *On the Origin of Species*. Written for non-specialists, it quickly attracted comment from scientists and scholars, but also quickly ignited a mainstream interest. Darwin was amazed to hear stories about his book flying off the shelves at Waterloo Station as commuters passed through. The more popular the book became, the more difficult it was for the establishment to ignore. Passions were roused and arguments began to rage. The most famous of these debates occurred at a routine "Botany and Zoology" meeting on 30 June 1860, when a crowd of more than 700 crammed themselves into a chamber at the Oxford University Museum. With many more listening outside unable to get in, the audience watched as Bishop Samuel Wilberforce lost his argument against evolution to Darwin's friend and supporter Thomas Huxley.

Darwin on man's abilities

In the last few pages of *Origin of Species*, Darwin alluded to the significance of his theory for Homo sapiens and, most importantly, the mental abilities that many consider set us apart from the rest of the animal kingdom. Darwin suggested that knowledge of how mental abilities were prehistorically acquired (i.e. evolved) could provide fundamental insight into the nature of these abilities (i.e. our psychology):

> In the distant future I see open fields for far more important researches. Psychology will be based on a new foundation, that of the necessary acquirement of each mental power and capacity by gradation. Light will be thrown on the origin of man and his history.

Note how Darwin emphasised gradualism as an important feature of this process of change. Gradualism is an enduring theme of evolutionary thinking – the idea that evolution proceeds in very small microevolutionary steps in terms of adaptations within a population. These small but observable changes can occur much more rapidly than the sort of timescales usually associated with geological time. Speciation – the arrival of a new species – is generally assumed to take longer but comes about through the accumulation of these small changes.

Generally, however, *Origin of Species* steered clear of discussing our own place in the evolutionary tale. Darwin was still stepping forward cautiously and provided no clear indication of what the light he alluded to would reveal. Addressing this question would be a challenge of the greatest sensitivity. Darwin's time was even more human-centred than our own. Holding the belief that humans were related to animals was, even leaving religion aside, commonly seen as a serious step along a slippery slope towards barbarism.

It was not long before Darwin felt forced to tackle this issue directly. Once again, he was prompted by Wallace but not, this time, because their ideas were converging. Within five years[7] of co-publishing views aligned with each other, Wallace began to get cold feet about evolution, as discussion began turning towards Homo sapiens. He started to distance himself from the notion that human abilities might have arisen through natural selection. Wallace was asking his readers, "How could 'natural selection', or survival of the fittest in the struggle for existence, at all favour the development of mental powers so entirely removed from the material necessities of savage men?" Now – with the theory of natural selection itself at stake – Darwin didn't hold back on relating evolutionary theory to Homo sapiens and society. Darwin responded to the question asked by Wallace in *The Descent of Man, and Selection in Relation to Sex*. Published in 1871, this book included discussion of evolutionary ethics and the differences between races and sexes. After drawing attention to similarities in the anatomy of humans and other animals, Darwin found intellectual similarities as well. He saw evidence of emotions in non-human animals such as curiosity, courage, affection and shame – feelings that have cultural significance in society, and also the stirrings of features considered distinctly human such as tool use, language, an appreciation of beauty and even religious inclinations. In beginning to plot a continuum between human and animal mental ability, he argued for an evolutionary basis for the arrival of our own species.

In Darwin's time, physical features could be measured but evidence for how mental abilities evolved was much more limited. Even today, there's much debate around how to compare the mental abilities of different species. Nevertheless, Darwin had made an important point: the theory of evolution could and should be applied to help understand our own brain. The leap from understanding a pepper moth's wing to human reasoning and learning may seem great, but the principle remains essentially the same. Understanding the evolutionary history of the pepper moth allows us to ask questions and learn more about how the wing colour of an existing moth "fits", or not, the environment it finds itself in (see box on pp. 6–7). Similarly, an evolutionary perspective on the brain may allow us to ask questions and learn more about how a modern human brain interacts with its environment, including its educational environment.

Evolution gets hijacked by notions of "progress"

Only a decade after publishing *Origin*, Darwin's half-cousin Galton was already using it to argue for a science of "eugenics". In Galton's own words, this was meant "to give to the more suitable races or strains of blood a better chance of prevailing speedily over the less suitable". Galton was interested in ways to manipulate and accelerate the processes by which human evolution was progressing, improving the fitness of the species by *artificial selection*. From its outset, the very definition of eugenics was a dangerous mixture of skewed morality and misinterpretation of science. Competition, as in one line of organisms adaptively advancing in their populations over another, was an observable fact that reflected the proposed mechanisms of natural selection. However, Galton was suggesting some fixed direction of progress that could be artificially accelerated. This was not part of Darwin's theory.

There is debate about whether Darwin believed evolution generally tended in a direction of something that could be called progress.[7] He was, after all, a man of his time, and a rosy notion of progress was central to the ethos of the British Empire. That said, Darwin's understanding of "fitness" did not lend itself well to the idea and he never associated himself with Galton's proposals. His statement in a letter to American palaeontologist Alpheus Hyatt appears to make his views clear: "After long reflection, I cannot avoid the conviction that no innate tendency to progressive development exists".[8]

Tragically, however, many influential people have been seduced by the idea that we are evolving in some identifiable direction of biological improvement, and that there is some advantage in accelerating humanity along it. At the beginning of the last century, the idea of eugenics began gathering supporters in many countries, amongst them well-respected politicians such as Winston Churchill and prominent biologists such as Charles Davenport. At first, eugenics found application in some relatively innocuous ways, such as marriage counselling. Ultimately, however, it became manifest in Hitler's programmes of extermination, justifying the pursuit of "racial hygiene".

Eugenics is dangerous because it parades a human notion of "progress" (which is defined by whoever is doing the parading) as something biologically defined. Darwin's own diaries reveal a deep wariness of human notions of progress. During his travels, he had journeyed through lands in the New World where efficient programmes of genocide were being conducted. He found himself meeting face-to-face with characters who were linked to dubious military operations such as General Rosas in Argentina. These meetings were necessary to gain permission to cross land where indigenous peoples were being corralled into a "Christian's zoo", where the Indian women "who appear above twenty years old are massacred in cold blood". Rather than expressions of wonder at the specimens accumulating in the hold, Darwin's most powerful emotional responses were reserved for the atrocities that were occurring around him. Darwin's family strongly adhered to the belief that slavery should be abolished, but these sentiments brought him into sharp conflict with the Beagle's captain. Such experiences may have sensitised Darwin to how ideas about difference can be exploited, encouraging him to emphasise the message of life's unity he saw in evolution. Indeed, it has been suggested that political and social issues, particularly slavery, were key driving forces for Darwin pursuing evolutionary theory with such tenacity.[9] Evolution is concerned with how one form of life changes into another and so suggests, as it did to Darwin, that all life derives from a common ancestor. The idea we are all part of the same slowly shifting web of life undermines any sense of fundamental difference between races (i.e. variations) within the same species. More broadly than this, it connects all species with one another, highlighting the interrelatedness of all life (see the tree of life opposite).

Modern evolutionary theory takes care to separate evolution from cultural notions of growth and improvement,[10] and to discourage any perception of progress in one direction or another. The evolutionary meaning of the term "fitness" does not imply a score on any simple scale (i.e. speed, size, etc.), but refers to the extent to which an organism, over generations, has become suited or "fitted" to the environment. Given the environment is itself subject to constant change, it is perhaps unsurprising that evolutionary change sustained in *any* one direction over time tends to be the exception rather than the rule.[11] Natural selection has sometimes been summed up as "survival of the fittest", but in recent years scientists have come to prefer "survival of the fit enough". Evolution favours those equipped to survive, but there are few prizes (and likely some costs) for having more equipment than is strictly needed. Further limitations on any alleged scientific basis for eugenics come from our modern understanding of genetics and human ability. It seems unlikely that traits for skills such as literacy and maths could easily be artificially selected for, since the same genes, in different combinations, contribute to high and low levels of these

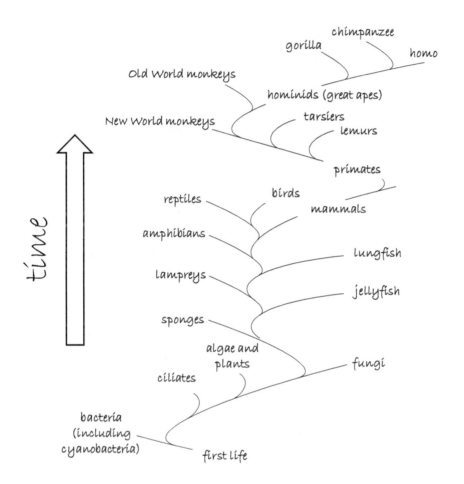

abilities. Nevertheless, we will see in Chapter 10 that modern science is making the idea of tinkering with human evolution much more possible.

The use of evolutionary theory to justify "scientific racism" has provided frightening examples of how science, authentic or otherwise, can be harnessed to seize moral authority when promoting ideas that are profoundly immoral. Eugenics remains a cautionary tale that reminds us of the importance of including ethical debate in the creation, interpretation and application of all science. Like many other powerful scientific ideas, evolutionary theory can be used for both good and evil, and how we use it should be informed by both science and by the views of those who might be affected. We will return to these issues again in Chapter 10.

Happily, modern evolutionary thinking has grandstanded more recently as a tool for encouraging racial tolerance rather than racial prejudice. South Africa is an example where this is particularly notable, since it was here that eugenics once played an influential role in supporting racist sentiment and justifying apartheid. In 1996, soon after the fall of the apartheid state, Mandela's government began to replace the old racially based system of education to reflect new values and principles for the country to aspire to. In the new curriculum, students would encounter concepts of evolution and particularly human evolution, so emphasising the common origin of humankind. The origin of humans from common ancestors was now per-ceived, as Darwin might have wished, as a strong unifying concept useful for building, rather than dividing, a racially diverse society.[12]

Evolution and genetics – the modern synthesis

Darwin's theory was founded on the idea that traits linked to survival and reproduction success could be inherited – and this fact could be clearly observed when he wrote and published his theory. But, in Darwin's day,

DNA and the processes by which traits are inherited

DNA is a very long molecule containing genetic instructions for the develop-ment, functioning and reproduction of an organism. It consists of two strands coiled around each other to form a double helix, divided up and packaged into separate pieces called chromosomes that are stored inside the nucleus of animal and plant cells.

During the growth and repair of an organism, the DNA copies itself before the cell divides to produce another cell, allowing the new cell to have an exact copy of the DNA that was in the old cell.

Also in the chromosome is ribonucleic acid (RNA), which helps put the DNA instructions into practice. The instructions in the DNA code for how a cell should produce proteins. Proteins do most of the work in cells and are critical for the structure, function and regulation of the body's tissues and organs, including brain tissue. Ultimately, these proteins will generate the biological structures that help create the appearance and behaviour of the whole organ-ism. A gene is a region of our DNA that codes instructions related to a trait. The most common human traits we think about (e.g. height and intelligence) are influenced by many such regions (i.e. they are polygenic). Traits are also, to a greater or lesser extent, influenced by environmental factors (e.g. nutrition and education).

Messenger RNA (mRNA) conveys the genetic information from the DNA to where molecular machines called ribosomes link amino acids together to no-one knew how such inheritance was happening. By 1865, Gregor Mendel published laws that showed how traits could be predictably inherited. Rediscovery of Mendel's ideas helped biologists in the 1930s to 1950s combine their observations with the new science of population genetics, creating the "modern synthesis", or "Neodarwinism". However, it was not until 1953 that the structure of deoxyribonucleic acid (DNA) and its role in storing genetic code were discovered, allowing the molecular processes of trait inheritance to finally be revealed (see box below).

By shedding light on the key process by which traits are inherited, modern genetics has supported the theory of evolution and helped us understand more about how it happens. For one thing, it seems clear that there must be sufficient genetic variation within a population for natural selection to work. This variation is essential for ensuring the presence of those with a markedly better fit, so enabling the traits associated with this fit to be selected. We now know the variation arises chiefly from the processes of

make the proteins. The amino acids are delivered by another type of RNA called transfer RNA (tRNA) but the order of linking is dictated by the mRNA, which follows the instructions it has carried from the DNA.

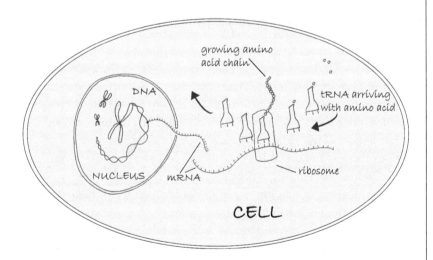

In sexual reproduction, DNA combines such that the offspring receive a novel mix of the DNA of their parents. This provides the genetic variation that makes evolution by natural selection possible.

genetic recombination which occur when organisms reproduce, but there are other factors contributing to this diversity too. These include processes of "mutation", in which a duplicate copy of an ancestral gene mutates and acquires a new function. This is not a very efficient source of improved fitness, because mutations appear more frequently to damage an organism than provide it with advantage. Even when competition and all else is equal, there will still be a small amount of randomness involved in how genes are transmitted across generations in a population. This "genetic drift" is another source of variation. These additional sources of variation are not adaptive in themselves: natural selection is still required for these changes to lead to improved fitness.

Natural selection is usually studied in terms of an organism surviving long enough to reproduce. However, sexual selection was also considered by Darwin as a process by which fitter traits might be selected for. Here, a mate is chosen for reproduction according to their fitness. The idea has a common-sense ring to it and feels credible, but concrete examples of sexual partners being chosen by fitness are only accumulating slowly.[13] Natural selection through being fit enough to survive, and so reproduce, remains the most widely applied theory of adaptation that improves the "fitness" of an organism, as coded in a population's genetic distribution.

Darwin, evolutionary theory and learning

There is a long history of evolution influencing educational thought. In 1881, Charles Darwin wrote a letter responding to the secretary of the Education Department of the American Social Science Association who had enquired about the significance of his theory for her area. In his letter, Darwin expresses his enthusiasm for understanding human development, and the need for research that could provide new insights. In his list of questions there is a sense that we should be concerned less with the objects of our children's attention, and more about the nature of their interaction with them. Darwin places emphasis on the importance of how the mental ability that underlies learning can be developed, rather than on the accumulation of specific knowledge and understanding. His ideas may reflect his own experience of pursuing his passion for collecting, in the face of little understanding from his father: "It may be more beneficial that a child should follow energetically some pursuit, of however trifling a nature, and thus acquire perseverance, than that he should be turned from it because of no future advantage to him".[14]

Perhaps, however, the most significant thing about Darwin's letter is that he doesn't provide specific suggestions on how we might teach and learn more effectively. Now a respected public figure, he had already expressed a very critical view of the school system, particularly its emphasis on the classics. He believed schools should broaden their curricula to include a greater range of subjects, notably science. When considering the relationship of evolutionary theory and education, Darwin did not use the opportunity to promote a list of changes that should be made. Instead, he believed his theory could be useful in identifying educationally relevant questions on human "mental and bodily development" and that these could prompt research that could produce educational insight. He seemed to be suggesting that educational change should arise from research that evolution can help frame, not directly from evolutionary theory itself.

Today this still seems wise advice – and perhaps timelier than ever. At this stage in the twenty-first century, we are just beginning to incorporate our new understanding of brain function and development into our ideas about how we teach and learn. Evolution cannot tell us how to teach and learn, but it can help us frame and understand this research. In this way, it can help us mentally digest the significance of our biology for revising our ideas about learning and the role of learning in who we are. Just as Darwin's theory prompted questions that helped us re-evaluate the relationship between a pepper moth's wing and the tree on which it rested, so the history of the learning brain may draw attention to new ways of thinking about learners and the environments in which they learn.

As the evolutionary story of the learning brain unfolds, you will see some familiar aspects of learning arriving over deep time. In each chapter, there will be some exploration of the links between these ancient processes and our own experience of learning as modern humans. Eventually we'll arrive in the present millennium and consider how the learning brain may evolve in the future. You'll have travelled several billion years by then and your own opinions about how we acquire knowledge and understanding may have changed – will human learning look different from a deep-time perspective? But enough jumping ahead; the story is about to begin . . .

2
ORIGINS

ABOUT 4.5 BILLION YEARS AGO a supernova exploded. Its wreckage was propelled into a nearby cloud of hydrogen gas and interstellar dust where, compressed by its own gravity, it formed our sun at its centre. Around this sun, a disc of leftover debris swirled. It was from this disc that the Earth and the other planets formed. To find out when the story of the learning brain began, we need to search here for learning in the earliest lifeforms we can find.

Being alive requires a constant struggle to maintain structure and order – an idea that many of us can relate to personally. But this is also true for the simplest of organisms, because all lifeforms must constantly work to maintain the natural order of their bodies. That requires taking in energy and resources from the surroundings and expelling the unwanted stuff. For animals, that's what commits us to the eat-and-excrete routine of daily life.

It's alive . . .

So, here we are in the primordial oceans that girdled a very young planet Earth (about 1 billion years old now). We are looking for a self-producing, self-repairing "thing" which draws in resources and energy from outside itself and flushes out its waste.

It's still a mystery how life began. Evolution helps explain what happened next, in terms of one species giving rise to another, but it is not a theory about the origins of life. In a letter to a friend, however, Darwin did speculate:

But if (and Oh! What a big if!) we could conceive in some warm little pond, with all sorts of ammonia and phosphoric salts, light, heat, electricity etc., present, that a protein compound was chemically formed ready to undergo still more complex changes.[15]

In other words, somehow, some non-living chemicals had to come together in the right combination to generate more complex ones such as amino acids, which in turn have the tendency to assemble themselves into longer strings.

In 1953, Stanley Miller and Harold Urey made their own warm little pond – applying electrical sparks (simulating lightning) to a primordial soup of hydrogen, methane, ammonia and steam, and found organic compounds forming such as amino acids.

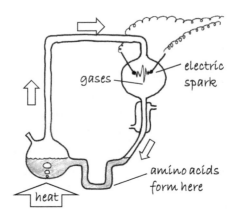

gases

electric spark

amino acids form here

heat

This experiment showed a warm little pond might have started things going, but this is not the only theory. For example, it has been suggested that life originated close to very hot hydrothermal vents in the deepest parts of the ocean, avoiding the need for a high-temperature atmosphere flooded with UV light and lightning bolts. Recently, tiny filaments and tubes formed by bacteria were discovered in Quebec and identified as the remains of microorganisms that lived at least 3.8 billion years ago in underwater hydrothermal vents.[16]

These remnants of earliest life would have been formed by prokaryotic organisms – single-celled bacteria without a cell nucleus.[17] The parts that a prokaryote needs to survive (proteins, DNA and energy-making bits) are packaged loosely inside the cell membrane, rather than in separate

The evolutionary clock has started ticking . . .

The timescales over which life has evolved are truly mind-boggling. To get some relative sense of the time periods involved, it can be helpful to shrink the whole story down to just 24 hours. Let's start out evolutionary clock ticking at **3.8 billion years ago** with these first signs of life (at the start of the new day – midnight) and stop it at the present time (at midnight when the day is over, 24 hours later). Look out for updates on the evolutionary clock at some key dates in the story, which will be in bold.

compartments. This is very different from their more complex descendants – the eukaryotes. The eukaryotic cell is much larger and more organised. Multicellular eukaryotes such as plants, fungi and animals, including ourselves, are made up of this sort of cell.

 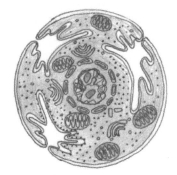

prokaryotic cell   eukaryotic cell

A third theory, however, proposes the building blocks of life arrived from outer space. Recently, the Rosetta spacecraft examined the dust and clouds around a comet and confirmed the presence of amino acids and other organic compounds suitable for making proteins. If life did come from space, then the range of timescales and possible scenarios for life's origins expands massively. And the mystery only deepens when we think about how life might first have spread. The Miller-Urey experiment was published in the same year as the discovery of DNA, and the new science of genetics raised a new question: how did the elaborate process of reproduction with DNA and RNA ever begin? Some scientists propose an RNA world in which RNA was not only able to store information but also replicated itself without any need for DNA or proteins. Others suggest something like life might have got started without DNA and RNA. They imagine "microspheres" subdividing into smaller ones, with each getting a portion of the bits required to keep taking in energy and outputting waste.

The mystery of life's origins shows no sign of being solved soon and the debates will rage on. Happily, however life started, there is at least some general agreement that our most ancient fossilized ancestor was a prokaryote. Despite being the simplest type of organism, the estimated number of different species of prokaryote existing now is a staggering 10 million to 1 billion different types. We owe them a lot. Prokaryotes, similar to existing cyanobacteria, helped shape the environment of our planet for future life. Cyanobacteria produce oxygen as a by-product of harvesting energy from sunlight (using the process known as photosynthesis). They group together in dense multi-layered mats in which hundreds of different species co-exist. Because of their tendency to trap sediment particles, these colonies form hard-layered structures called stromatolites. Evidence of stromato-

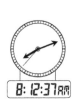

lites has been found from as early as **2.5 billion years ago**,[18] but they may have been pumping oxygen into the air for at least another billion years before that.[19] Modern stromatolites sometimes appear as semi-submerged mushroom-shaped rocks in very salty lakes or lagoons, where the saltiness protects them from over-grazing by snails and sea-urchins:

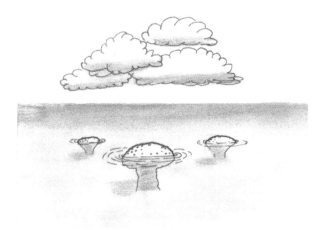

So prokaryotes are very wonderful – but can we really find anything to do with learning in a one-cell organism so primitive that its precious bits are all mixed up in one bag?

Memory: remembering and acting on the past

Amazingly, even in this most primitive of organisms, we do find something we can call learning. Prokaryotes, like all organisms, face the challenge that their world can change. Even if all else remains the same, just an organism's habit of harvesting local resources will change its environment. At its most basic, learning can be about detecting these changes, because it means comparing the world now with the way it was a while ago – which means some memory of the old world must be stored somewhere.

Cyanobacteria rely on being supplied by the nutrient phosphate to survive and grow, but they live in conditions where this varies greatly – often in "pulses". Since there are times when no phosphate is available, they need to take it up and store it during a pulse – but must avoid gorging so much that it stops their cells working properly.[20] Cyanobacteria can't feel or sense how much phosphate they have already consumed but, somehow, they do seem to remember it. Former changes in uptake of phosphate inform new changes, resulting in just the right amount for healthy growth.

Scientists are still trying to work out how cyanobacteria remember, but memory in another type of prokaryote has been much more studied. *E. coli* is a prokaryote with a bad reputation, but it provides a good example of how even the simplest form of life can achieve a simple type of learning.

E. coli – a primordial student

Not all *E. coli* are bad for you, and benign types exist in our gut in vast numbers. In terms of information, like their human host, the key input for an *E. coli* is sensory data arriving from the outside world and the key output is movement. They can move by rotating a set of filaments (their flagella) like a propeller. When *E. coli* rotate their flagella clockwise, the filaments work together as one and the cell moves forward. When they rotate them anti-clockwise, the filaments become uncoordinated and the cell "tumbles" randomly around. So, there are really only two travel options for an *E. coli* – forward or tumble:

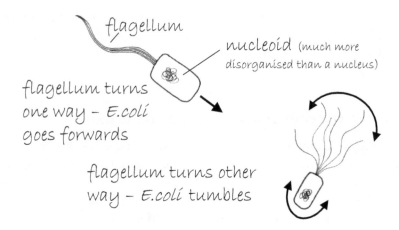

flagellum

nucleoid (much more disorganised than a nucleus)

flagellum turns one way – E.coli goes forwards

flagellum turns other way – E.coli tumbles

How an *E. coli* remembers using chemicals

An *E. coli* experiences the outside world through a range of different types of *receptors* in its membrane. These are activated when particular types of chemical occupy them. Some of these receptors respond to nourishing nutrients that feed the *E. coli*. When not occupied, these receptors can send a chemical message to the flagella making it more likely they will change rotation and the *E. coli* will tumble. However, the *E. coli* really only wants to tumble if the food supply is worse than it was – rather than just continuing to be poor.

The cell's memory for the past is recorded in the nutrient receptors themselves. When a nutrient receptor becomes occupied, it attaches a methyl group to remind itself:

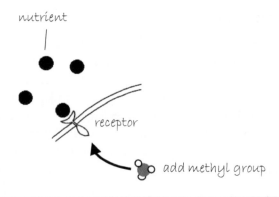

nutrient

receptor

add methyl group

The way an *E. coli* employs these options depends on whether things are getting better (go forward) or worse (tumble). This means it can detect how the world outside is changing, which requires remembering what the world was like a few moments ago. In other words, it can learn. It achieves this by having receptors that, when activated by chemicals in the outside world, store a methyl group as a record of the event (see box below).

Prokaryotes and learning

So, it appears that even a humble *E. coli* – with its one cell and disorderly innards – can direct itself towards a goal based on previous experience. It has a "memory" – but can we really call it learning? Certainly, the words

If a receptor becomes unoccupied while holding a methyl group, then it means things have just got worse – so it sends a chemical tumble signal and drops its methyl group:

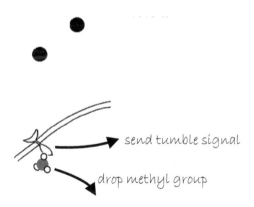

Once unoccupied *and* not holding a methyl group, it doesn't carry on sending a tumble message – because this just means times are bad – but not necessarily worse than they were. A similar mechanism involves receptors that detect toxins, allowing the *E. coli* to tumble when poisons that might damage it are increasing.

"memory" and "learning" are often used interchangeably in neurobiology reports, but most educators would say there's a difference. Educators usually think about learning as a process involving social interaction in the classroom.[21] In education, there is also great emphasis placed on the "higher" levels of learning (e.g. understanding how to analyse, synthesise and evaluate) compared to rote learning of facts and figures. However, memory is a common factor on which *all* the types of learning depend – whether we are talking about rote learning, mathematical concepts or even the social construction of morality though dialogue. So, although learning is not just about memory, memory is an essential part of its foundation. Incredibly, this ability may have been present in the earliest types of lifeform that existed on our planet.

And there is another, more fundamental principle that *E. coli* demonstrate that is essential for understanding why the brain is relevant to learning and education: whenever learning occurs, there *must* be a biological mechanism that makes it possible. This is as true for *E. coli* as it is for us. Understanding our own biological mechanisms can help us understand how we can learn.

Eukaryotes

Around **1.6 billion years ago** the first eukaryotes show their presence. These were still single-celled organisms, but they were bigger, boasted a nucleus and their other important bits were packaged in an orderly fashion. The functioning parts of an eukaryote may have initially been created through a process of *symbiosis*, in which some prokaryotes were effectively absorbed inside others, transferring most of their genome to the host cell along the way. Echoes of the simple chemical signal system appear to have been transferred in this process. However, the increased complexity of a eukaryote allowed for more sophisticated types of signalling, including the use of hormones and hormone-like substances such as pheromones.

Some of the closest living relatives of the first eukaryotes, which would still have been single-celled, support something called *associative learning* – i.e. learning to associate two previously unrelated things. This makes some impressive learning behaviours possible. *Spirostomum*, for example, is a single-celled living eukaryote found in fresh water and salt water. It can learn which approaches to mating are associated with success, and so choose the ones that produce the best outcomes. Learning has a high profile in the rituals by which these organisms get together and exchange their genetic material. This suggests learning influences whose genetic material is communicated to the next generation, and so can play an important role in a population's evolution. If mating and learning were intertwined like this in earlier eukaryotes, this would have accelerated the rate at which new adaptations for learning evolved.

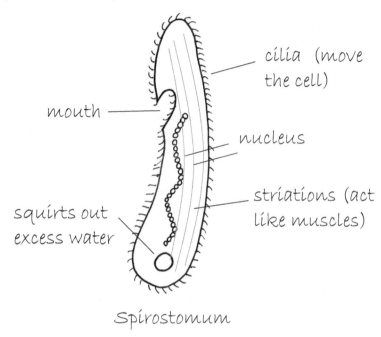

mouth

cilia (move the cell)

nucleus

striations (act like muscles)

squirts out excess water

Spirostomum

The courtship rituals of *Spirostomum* involve contact but also feature avoiding contact through contraction and reversing the cilia that power them along.[22]

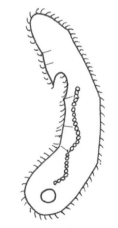

A spirostomum does a contraction

Fitter versions of this organism take a flashy approach to advertising themselves by playing hard to get with more frequent contractions. This is an expensive strategy in terms of energy, but it can arouse their mate and make success more likely in that way. In contrast, less fit organisms usually take a more prudent approach. They increase their chances of success by conserving energy and making themselves more available, with reduced contractions.

An individual *Spirostomum* learns to combine these two strategies of flashiness and prudence to maximise their chances of success. For example, an unfit organism will learn to be occasionally flashy, if being flashy is producing such success that it justifies using the little energy it has. More impressively, if an unfit organism finds itself sandwiched between a flashy peer and a potential mate, then it can sometimes learn to "hack into" their rival's contraction-reversal signals. The less-fit *Spirostomum* can use these signals to encourage their own conjugation with the target mate, after this target has become aroused by the fitter competitor.

These single-celled organisms can receive each other's vibrations through *ion channels* that exist in their cell membrane. When these channels activate, they let in charged particles called ions. In this way, ion channels can code the sense of vibration into an electrical signal that can be communicated across the cell. This electrical transmission of information is an important innovation that would have implications for higher lifeforms, and it has been studied in another single-celled eukaryote called *Paramecium*.[23]

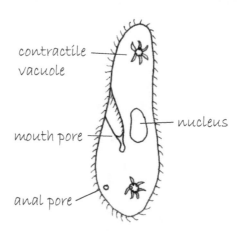

Paramecium thrives in stagnant dirty ponds and generally swims forward until it bangs into something. Then it will momentarily reverse and move forward again, inevitably in a slightly different direction. This happens because the calcium ion channels in its membrane open on impact. This allows positively charged calcium ions to flow in, giving the cell a brief positive charge. This positive charge causes all the cilia to change the direction of their beating, driving the organism into reverse. Each opening of the calcium ion channels also opens other channels which allow positive ions to pass out, helping the cell to return to its original electrical state. So, *Paramecium* basically turns a physical collision into a momentary electrical pulse that gets transmitted across the cell, allowing all the cilia to reverse together. This is shown on the highly stylised diagram of a Paramecium below, which shows a few of the receptors involved and only one of its many cilia:

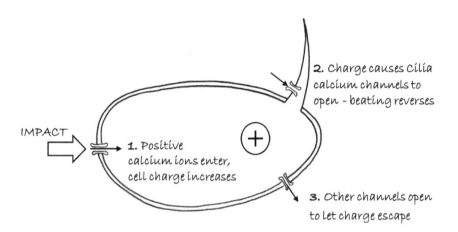

This usually solves the problem of getting past whatever obstruction was in front. However, *Paramecium* can also learn when short periods of backward swimming are not working and longer periods of going backwards are needed. Its ion channels open for longer after several impacts in a row, which indicates the obstruction is not shifting and more backward swimming is necessary.[24] It could be argued this is a primitive type of associative learning – the *Paramecium* is associating the obstruction with difficulty in moving forwards and is modifying its approach accordingly.

Evolution of a mechanism to turn sensory information into momentary pulses of electricity was to have great implications for more complex forms of life. Although we are multicellular, we are composed of cells with nuclei and so we are also categorised, along with plants, fungi and all other animals, as eukaryotic. Indeed, like the humble *Paramecium*, the first step that enables sensory information to enter our bodies is this conversion into electrical pulses. There is also another pattern already emerging. All three microbes that we have looked at convert incoming sensory information into outgoing movement information. "Sense-into-action" will become an organising principle of all the many different types of nervous system we will encounter in our history of the learning brain, including our own.

Microbes such as *E. coli* are so small that you could fit many billions of them into a single drop of water, and yet each can learn about the world and act on the memory of it a few moments later. Even more surprisingly, amongst these relatives of early life that swarm around us, we find the beginnings of processes, principles and patterns that would one day play a vital role in our own learning brain. We could not learn anything today without ion channels, receptors and electrical signalling, yet scientists believe these have existed for well over a billion years.

Multicellular organisms

Multicellular organisms are thought to have evolved from single-celled ancestors with flagella coming together in colonies, possibly taking the shape of hollow spheres.[25] If you are a cell, sticking together can mean better chances of survival for you and also for any of your genetic mutations that help you achieve this feat. This way, it's easy to imagine how multicellular life got started. One of the big advantages is defence. Being part of a big cell cluster makes you more resistant to predatory cells. You are less exposed because some of your sides are joined to those of others. Also, it can result in more efficient use of nutrients. For example, clumps of yeast cells share the substance they secrete to digest the nutrients around them. Single yeast cells cannot survive in low-nutrient conditions because they are unable to share the workload of digesting.[26] However, getting together with other cells is not all plain sailing.

Sponges and the first animals

Going multicellular has its drawbacks. For one for thing, even when just two cells get together, it can make movement difficult because each must coordinate their movement with the other. Think how difficult we can find coordinating our movements in a three-legged race. Then imagine the complexity of coordinating movement across hundreds and thousands of cells in an organised way. Little surprise, then, that we find a tendency towards a more sedentary life amongst our most ancient of multicellular ancestors: the sponge. Nevertheless, this multicellular organism does move and this quality helps the sponge qualify as a true animal. Although adult sponges stick in one place, they must still feed on the nutrients they filter out of the water that flows through them. This makes it important for them to coordinate some simple movements over their bodies. These include contracting to squeeze out materials that might block this vital water flow, and cells achieve this coordination through simple chemical signalling. We also find some movement in the early stages of a young sponge developing. When the eggs of modern sponges hatch, larvae emerge which comprise balls of cells able to transport themselves using their flagella or cilia that are attached to their outer layer. The larvae swim for a few days before settling. The early ability of sponge larvae to move, although limited, allows the species to spread more readily and makes it more likely to survive.

Despite the challenges of coordinated movement, multicellularity does allow for the possibility of cells within the same organism doing different jobs. We see this in the sponge when, as the larvae settle, cells transform themselves into the different types that a small-scale sponge needs to start out – cells for drawing in water, for pores, for closing pores, for carrying nutrients and for their hard structure:

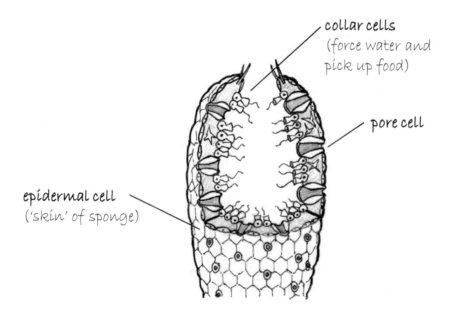

collar cells
(force water and
pick up food)

pore cell

epidermal cell
('skin' of sponge)

Soon, the advantages of this specialisation, such as allowing the development of different organs specialised in different functions, would open the door to a vast range of multicellular solutions to the problems of how to survive in different environments. This specialisation of cells would also help solve the problem of coordinating movement.

At around 635 Myr, we see an explosion of strange (Ediacaran) forms in the fossil record. These may represent the first multicellular animals but they seem so remote from the lifeforms we know today that we have no real idea whether they moved or not. Given the coordination challenge of multicellular moving, it seems likely that the first animals were, like the sponge, not very mobile. Fossils we can clearly identify as sponges date from **600 Myr**.[27]

The arrival of the neuron and the brainless jellyfish

For animals to really take off, the movement problem would have to be solved. Directional movement had already existed amongst single-celled organisms for a long time before sponges arrived, emphasising its advantages for avoiding danger and finding food. Multicellularity clearly also had benefits, even if it meant being a sponge and tied to a rock all your adult life – but a multicellular animal that could move more readily would have the best of both worlds, being able to occupy habitats and obtain food that a tethered sponge just can't reach.

But what – hypothetically – would it take to make a sponge walk? A walking sponge would need a fast, efficient flow of information between its cells. The response of one set of cells would have to be rapidly informed by the response of others, and by information from the environment about where the sponge wants to go and how well it's getting there. All this data would need to be orchestrated to move the whole organism in the right direction. Multicellularity may have created this problem but, through its potential to produce specialised cells, it also helped the solution evolve. This solution was a cell dedicated to information processing: the neuron. This cell can pass its momentary electrical pulse down a long "axon" to terminals that can connect to other cells, allowing information to be networked across the organism.

All neurons follow the same basic plan shown here (although an important difference is that the axons of humans and other vertebrates are usually covered in myelin, which insulates and increases the speed of transmission):[28]

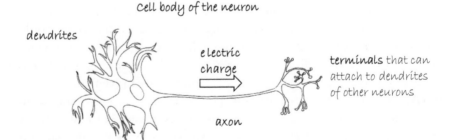

Cell body of the neuron

dendrites

electric charge

terminals that can attach to dendrites of other neurons

axon

As early as **560 Myr** ago we find the first fossil evidence of jellyfish[29] swimming in the oceans. These are the earliest multicellular animals we know were on the move, and so we can assume the neuron has arrived. Multicellular life was now in possession of something we can call a nervous system – a set of interconnected neurons or neural network. Jellyfish largely owe their superb swimming abilities to this system. They achieve their movement through the oceans by radially expanding and contracting to push the water behind them, but do so with expert timing – making them the world's most efficient swimmers.[30] For a multicellular animal, the type of coordinated movement required to achieve such a feat requires monitoring where the different parts of one's body are and transforming this information into instructions about what each part should do next. The nervous system of the jellyfish does this processing continuously and at a very high speed. How does this happen?

How a jellyfish can swim

The neuron cells we find in the nervous system of all modern animals, including jellyfish, operate with many of the processes present in the earlier lifeforms, such as membrane receptors, electrical pulses and ion channels. However, unlike those primitive organisms, every creature with a nervous system has a complete set of these processes in every one of its many neurons, with each neuron able to connect with other neurons to form a complex system for information transfer. The electrical impulse that jellyfish (and human) neurons use to communicate is created by the opening of sodium channels. This discharge of electricity can happen when the dendrites of the neuron are stimulated by the output of another neuron. The pulse then travels down the stimulated neuron's axon and, in a jellyfish, the electric charge travels across a connection (or synapse) to reach the dendrites of another neuron, allowing information to pass very rapidly from one neuron to the next.

A simple nervous system might comprise a network of neurons. Special neurons can convert a sensory event (such as touch, vision, sound) into the first set of pulses and so provide an initial input to the system. The strength of a signal from a neuron is represented by the rate at which its pulses are firing off. The signal then gets passed through the network to output neurons, which may convert the incoming signal into a muscular response. Even in a simple example of such a network, the neurons can all be highly interconnected with each other, meaning an input signal is getting processed into an output across many routes at once. Each connection (or synapse) encountered by the signal along each route can potentially reduce or amplify the strength of the signal before it reaches the next neuron, which is also receiving and adding in outputs from other ones. It is the efficiency "setting" of each connection (how much comes out compared with how much goes in) that defines what an input gets turned into. With the correct settings, a piece of sensory information (e.g. where your finger is now) gets turned into the appropriate output action (how your finger should move next).

Our brain is often compared to a computer but actually this "parallel processing" across many routes is very different to how most computers work. Computers tend to operate by following a step-by-step plan that could be described using a flowchart. In contrast, information in a neural network flows through the various pathways in the network simultaneously, with the efficiency of each connection (or synapse) making only a small contribution to how the input signal gets transformed into an output. One advantage of this is called "redundancy" – you can cut out some of the routes and the network may still give something like the original output. So, if a small percentage of neurons die, or connections are damaged, the network may not work so well but it will probably still work. This "graceful degradation" contrasts greatly with what happens when a line of code becomes corrupted in your computer. If one part of the sequence stalls, the whole process crashes. For similar reasons, if there's something corrupted or odd about the input, the network may not completely fail and can still produce a sensible output. This is how the structure of our own brains help us guess at identifying objects, words and faces, even when we haven't seen anything exactly like them before.

That said, there are some big differences between jellyfish networks and our own. For one thing, strictly speaking, a jellyfish doesn't have a brain. Their neurons are not clustered together with a centre that qualifies as a central nervous system. Instead, their neurons are distributed radially around their bodies – close to where sensing and response are required:

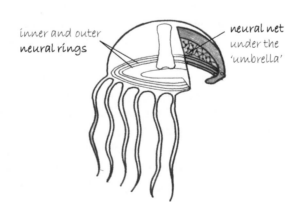

inner and outer
neural rings

neural net
under the
'umbrella'

The grace with which jellyfish swim is also helped by how quickly information gets passed across their neural connections but, for the most part, their synapses work quite differently to our own. Between most jellyfish neurons, information is passed electrically across the small gap that separates the end of one neuron's axon terminal from the dendrite of the next. The impressive speed of this electrical synapse makes it perfect for supporting superbly fast and coordinated movements. Jellyfish swim expertly downwards to avoid unsalty water, dive in response to turbulence, avoid walls of rock, collect together in swarms and maintain a particular direction when swimming.[31] They seem very skilful at transforming "sense-into-action".

However . . . there is a drawback to having the nervous system of a jellyfish, and this becomes clear when we look at their learning abilities.

Jellyfish can learn – to some extent, anyway. *Aurelia labiate*, for example, is a type of moon jellyfish found in the Northern Pacific amongst estuaries, small bays, lagoons and rocky shores. These are complex changing environments with a variety of hazards that include tides, jagged rocks and edges of shells, submerged tree branches and changing sources of prey. Here, the waters tend to change in terms of temperature, saltiness and oxygen content. The neural networks of this jellyfish usually help it swim down to avoid unsalty water, and swim up when it bumps into something – but what happens when things get more complicated? Can jellyfish learn to change their ways if, when trying to swim down to avoid low saltiness, they also keep bumping into something? A recent study showed that after a third bump, jellyfish spend less time swimming up than they did after the first or second bump and some of them may swim sideways.[32] In other words, some *are* learning that this has happened before and *are* changing their behaviour accordingly. They are associating their previous strategy with failure to escape the bumping. Their alternative strategy suggests some sort of rewiring of the connections in the nervous system has occurred – resulting in the same bump now producing a different movement. But that is about the limit of their learning ability. A jellyfish has trouble outshining a single-celled *Paramecium* in terms of changing its behaviour, despite being a much larger, multicellular animal with a nervous system. This is because learning for any animal means the efficiency of the connections between its neurons must be able to change, enabling the network to generate a new output for the same input. Most of the neural connections of a jellyfish have not evolved to easily change in this way. Their brain is, to a large extent, hard-wired, i.e. their connections are fixed in a way that is passed down through generations.

We should try not to be rude about jellyfish. They may be poor students, but they have what they need to survive within their own niche. They have inhabited our planet for over 20 times longer than we have, and their enduring (and presently increasing) numbers demonstrate their huge success as a species. What's more, jellyfish do have some synapses that are more amenable to learning, but their lifestyle means they don't need many of them. The more elaborate nature of this other type of synapse means its efficiency can be changed in lots of different ways, so supporting a much richer range of learning processes. This is the chemical synapse, and it's the neural connection that would eventually dominate the brains of most other animals and all mammals, including humans.

The chemical synapse

For learning to occur, we need a brain whose connectivity can be changed – i.e. a brain with a set of connections that are "plastic". The chemical synapse is thought to have evolved alongside the electrical one, but it was a connection with much more learning potential. At a chemical synapse, an electrical pulse

How a chemical synapse works

The terminals (or ends) of an axon contain chemicals referred to as "neuro-transmitters" enclosed in small spheres known as vesicles. On the other side of a small gap are the dendrites of the next neuron which are waiting to receive the neurotransmitters.

When the electrical pulse arrives down the axon to the terminals of a neuron, the membrane depolarises and causes ion channels to open that let in calcium ions (sound familiar? – see p. 29). This forces packets of the neuro-transmitter to move towards the membrane, where calcium-sensitive proteins attached to the vesicles are activated. These proteins change shape, causing the packets touching the membrane to fuse with it, open up and dump their neurotransmitter into the gap. The amount of chemical that gets dumped depends on the extent to which the transmitting neuron was electrically acti-vated. Some of the neurotransmitter that gets dumped is just lost, but some of it travels across and occupies receptors for that neurotransmitter on the other side. What happens next depends on the type of neurotransmitter/receptor, and it can make the firing of the next neuron more or less likely. *How much* more likely, or less likely, depends on the efficiency of this process – i.e. the efficiency of the synapse. It is this efficiency that changes when we learn.

arriving at the end of one neuron's axon causes a chemical to be released and cross the gap to the dendrite of the next neuron. Receiving a chemical signal can cause the next neuron to do a variety of things, including produce its own electrical pulse (see box on this page). This coding of an electrical signal into a chemical and then back again may seem a rather indirect way to send a message between neurons. However, this momentary conversion of information into chemicals means it is much more amenable to getting involved with other brain processes. These include processes that can change the efficiency of the synapse – or so-called "synaptoplasticity".

Synaptoplasticity

How can a network "learn" to change the output it produces for a given input? At a neural level, this can happen if, *as a result of one neuron helping to fire another neuron*, the efficiency of the connection between the two neurons is increased.[33] This effect is sometimes expressed by the phrase "neurons that fire together wire together". It was first observed in the brain tissue of rabbits, when scientists applied brief high-frequency electrical

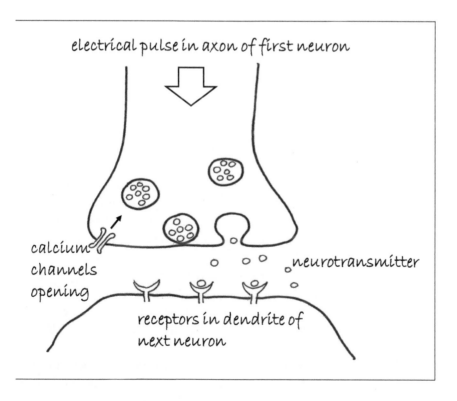

electrical pulse in axon of first neuron

calcium channels opening

neurotransmitter

receptors in dendrite of next neuron

stimulation to synapses, and showed that this caused a persistent strengthening in their firing rate.[34] This phenomenon, known as long-term potentiation (LTP), is now generally accepted as the most convincing cellular basis for learning and memory. It has also since been studied in animals that are only distantly related to vertebrates, such as the octopus, suggesting LTP is an ancient learning mechanism.[35,36] However, the differences in underlying LTP mechanisms across species suggest that it has arisen on many different occasions, and in different ways, throughout our evolutionary history.[37]

This might already seem an elaborate process, but things can get much more complicated. For example, some neurotransmitters are received by receptors that do not directly affect the firing of the next neuron, but instead send out other chemical messages that influence the neuron's response to other neurotransmitters – so-called secondary messages. This complexity is a bit daunting – but it underlies the diversity of mechanisms required for a sophisticated brain that can learn in so many ways.

How did that ever happen?

Given that most of evolution is supposed to be very gradual, how could something as complex as a chemical synapse evolve in small, slow stages? This question has perplexed scientists and is one reason why, originally, electrical synapses were thought to have evolved first, and then developed into chemical ones. However, you might remember we have already come across receptors and ion channels in the simpler forms of life from which jellyfish evolved. This "platform" for evolving chemical synapses has been particularly studied in Choanoflagellates which, in genetic terms, appear to be the closest single-celled relative of multicellular animals that is alive today. They are very like the feeding cells of sponges, possessing a single flagellum that moves around to trap food inside their collar. Although they do not possess anything like a synapse, they already have many of the key elements required. These include channels equivalent to the calcium ion channels we find in synapses, and the use of complex proteins that are also needed for the fusion, opening and dumping of packets of neurotransmitters through the cell membrane.[38] It appears, then, that some important building blocks existed long before the arrival of the neuron, with increasing complexity gradually giving rise to a chemical synapse.[39]

If the chemical synapse did evolve in small numbers in jellyfish, they were never going to multiply and become part of an impressive learning system – simply because jellyfish don't need to learn that much. Instead, another evolutionary development and a wholly new type of animal would create the demand for more complex learning and the plasticity that supports it. This new development was forward motion.

Arrival of the bilaterals – and the brain

Jellyfish have no front or back end. Their radial symmetry means they have no commitment to move in any one direction. However, such a commitment offered opportunities to evolve in new ways. It meant an organism could become more organised and streamlined for speed in that one direction, turning its body to escape from peril or rush towards food. The dedication to direction also led to bilateral symmetry, with sensing gear focused towards the direction and target of travel. If you have direction, there are some other parts of your body that are better at the designated front end, such as your mouth, so you can eat on arrival. This leads to your front end being a good place to cluster the neurons involved with your senses and movement too – since there's now a greater chance

---

Embodied cognition and the enactment effect

Theories of "embodied cognition" emphasise how the learning capacities of humans (like those of all bilaterians, and even jellyfish and some bacteria) evolved to convert sensory input into movement output. On this basis, we might expect better learning when knowledge is embodied in meaningful movements, such as gestures that are relevant to the learning. Many studies confirm this "enactment effect" in children and adults, and studies of brain imaging indicate greater activation of brain regions for sensing and movement as a likely explanation.[40] This effect has potential applications in the classroom. This was demonstrated in a recent intervention in which four-year-old Greek children were taught new animal names in English.[41] The children were taught with flashcards that showed the name in English and Greek (e.g. "Σκύλος–Dog") and all children were asked to repeat the name when they saw the card. In a second group, children also gestured like the animal, and in a third group they gestured and acted like the animal. Gesturing improved learning, and gesturing and acting further improved it.

Numerous other examples of the enactment effect include improvements in an adult memory test of action phrases when these were performed,[42] the benefits for recall and understanding when 8–11-year-olds traced temperature graphs on iPads with their fingers[43] and the benefits for young children's knowledge of two-digit numbers when they "stepped" through the numbers that they said out loud.[44]

of getting nibbled at your back end – where you have less sensory gear for alerting you to predators. For these straightforward reasons, bilateralism arrived alongside a gathering of neurons at the front end, i.e. something like a central nervous system, or brain.

If you're going to have a direction of travel, you also have new problems that this central nervous system must solve, such as the critical issue: where should you go? Making this decision would often be a matter of life and death, so having a plastic brain that can learn from experience was a huge advantage. For bilaterians, the role of learning movement in our evolutionary history and the "sense-to-action" principle has been a huge driver of our brain evolution. So much so that many think it unwise to consider human mental processes involving reasoning and memory as separable from those involving action. The idea that our thoughts are "embodied" in an action-based nervous system helps us understand the "enactment" effect in human learning (see box on the previous page).

The first bilaterian?

Bilaterians (including ourselves) are assumed to have originally evolved from radially symmetrical creatures with the type of neural networks found in jellyfish. The closest living creature to the first bilaterian is thought to be the humble flatworm. Flatworms have primitive eyes and sensors for detecting changes in nutrients and toxins,[45,46] as well as electric[47] and magnetic fields.[48,49] This rich variety of sensory information is processed by their nervous system into a complex set of behaviours that allows them to navigate and exploit their world. At their front end are two clusters of neurons (ganglia) that operate like a simple brain, and may resemble the beginnings of the vertebrate brain:[50]

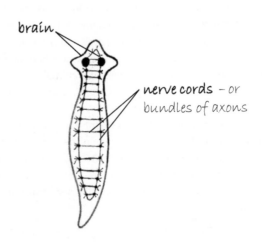

brain

nerve cords – or bundles of axons

Most of the types of neurotransmitter that have been discovered in our brain can also be found in the nervous system of a flatworm.[51,52] However, the flatworm has only around 10,000 neurons (that's about a ten-millionth of our own stock).[53] Nevertheless, flatworms can learn in some interesting ways. For example, they can decide to avoid a piece of fish (potential food) after it becomes associated with potential danger – such as being next to some mashed-up flatworms. They will even continue to avoid this food later, when the evidence of damaged flatworms has been removed. This is not a trivial challenge, because the speed at which a flatworm learns this association must be just right. If a worm learns avoidance at the merest hint of danger, they miss out on a lot of good food for no reason, while learning too slowly may result in death and disaster. The learning itself requires that connections must change their efficiency such that the smell of the fish produces an avoidance response rather than approach. After a few fishy encounters with the danger association, the plasticity of chemical synapses allows this rewiring to take place.

There is much, however, that remains to be understood about the details of how flatworms learn. For example, it seems clear that some part of what they learn must be stored outside of what we might call their brain. If a flatworm is decapitated after training, it can grow a new head (and brain) and still show evidence of having retained what it learnt prior to decapitation.[54] This has prompted many studies seeking the mechanisms by which neurons, and their memories, might be restored for human benefit.[55]

The great explosion of animal life

The oldest fossil that has been confidently identified as bilateral dates from 555 Myr. It has been named Kimberella and appears as a pear-shaped animal

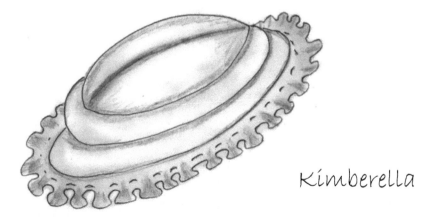

Kimberella

that grew to at least 14 cm long. Like most fossils of this age, its dissimilarity from known lifeforms makes it difficult to know much more about it.

It is generally believed that Kimberella, and the two great categories of animals we have today, all evolved from those small crawling worms that first boasted a brain. One of these great categories would include molluscs and insects and the other would include the vertebrates (such as fishes, reptiles, birds and mammals). The learning of all these animals would benefit from a central system of neurons highly interconnected with chemical synapses.

3

THE VERTEBRATE BRAIN

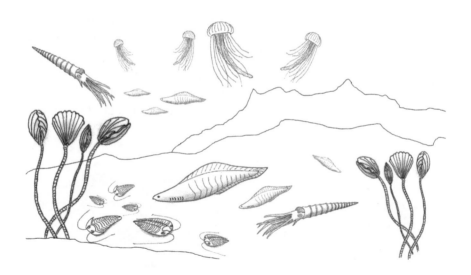

IF YOU WERE SWIMMING in the oceans around **542 Myr**, a hugely diverse range of lifeforms would be swimming around you: you're experiencing the "Cambrian explosion" of life. Some of these lifeforms might even seem a bit familiar, because the body plans of Cambrian creatures mostly resemble those of modern ones. You might spot molluscs, brachiopods, echinoderms, trilobites and, importantly for our own evolution, one of the first vertebrates: the jawless fish.

20:34:36 PM

The stage is now set for a grand evolutionary event: the colonisation of the land by animals – but it doesn't happen suddenly.

Serious migration to the land could never have happened at all unless the land had begun to offer its own food. Fortunately for the first settlers, the land had been supporting microbial life for over 2 billion years. These microbes were helping to gradually transform the land with nutrients. In other news, an oxygen-loving eukaryote had managed to absorb cyanobacteria,[56–59] with its ability for photosynthesis. This had given rise to green algae – a hugely significant arrival because all plant life would evolve from it. Indeed, out of the now crowded Cambrian seas, primitive plants were now evolving to thrive on land – benefiting greatly from the space to collect more sunlight. We find fossilised spores – the first signs of plants – in rocks dated to around 470 Myr.[60] Feeding off the plants, and off each other, came the insects, worms and snails.

Another type of organism, the vertebrate, was also working up to the leap from water to land. Actually, we shouldn't use the word "leap", because our evolutionary principles suggest we must imagine a gradual process. Most likely, small modifications helped some creatures enjoy longer excursions out of the water, enabling them to feed and breed in the mud, even though their lifestyle was still, essentially, water-based. This tendency towards spells of land-based life can still be seen today in the Queensland lungfish. This is a fish whose primitive lungs help it survive several days out of water and whose family has a left a fossil record going back beyond 400 Myr:[61,62]

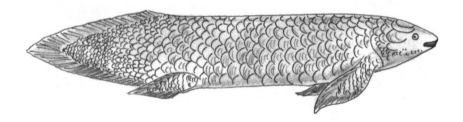

Apart from the equipment for breathing, ocean animals moving out of the water also needed transport. Some already had most of the basic kit required since, based on recent finds in Poland, marine fish were walking along the ocean floor by 395 Myr.[63] Different forms of early four-footed animals are found from about 375 Myr, but these creatures would not have been able to stray far inland.[64–66] Like all amphibians, they would have laid their eggs in the water, and being close to the water was a critical issue that put a limit on their land-based wanderings. The last tether to water was finally broken when an egg evolved with its own amniotic fluid and a hard-enough shell to survive a dry nest. Now, animals could spend their whole life cycle roaming a land that was increasingly full of lush vegetation and forests.

Eggs have a very low chance of surviving the fossilisation process[67] so it's difficult to know when animals that didn't lay eggs in water first arrived (i.e. the so-called "amniotes") first arrived. However, by around **300 Myr**, we do see two great groups of these vertebrates fully adapted to life on land. Some of these are vegetarian and able to take full and direct advantage of the plant life and, as part of the food chain, pass it on to their meat-eating predators.[68] One of these amniotic groups gave rise to modern mammals and the other group were the reptiles, from which birds would also evolve. For well over a hundred million years, the dinosaurs dominated the land and air. Evidence of mammals is only found from **225 Myr**, with the arrival of a mammal-like animal called *Adelobasileus*:

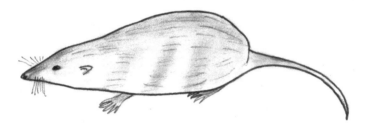

The vertebrate ground plan

All existing and extinct vertebrates (including reptiles, mammals, birds and, of course, ourselves) evolved from the jawless fish. This explains why we all share the same basic brain layout, and also possess the same set of basic learning processes. The "tripartite" ground plan for the brain has been retained for over half a billion years, and in a general form might be represented something like this:[69]

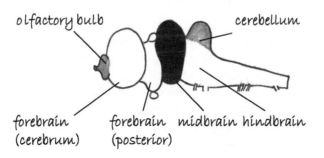

There are three key parts (explaining the "tri" in "tripartite"). These consist of the forebrain (to which is attached the olfactory bulb – important for smell), the midbrain and hindbrain (including the cerebellum). What varies greatly with different species is the relative size of the different parts. This variation reflects how brains have evolved to support the mental abilities required to survive in whatever environment they have adapted to – i.e. their "niche" (see box below).

The learning needs of vertebrates on land bore some resemblance to those of their relatives they had left behind in the ocean. They needed to organise information by association, to finely adjust their movement, to seek out food and to recall something of what happened yesterday. These are different types of learning that are served by four distinct learning systems already possessed, to a greater or lesser extent, by their fishy ancestors. However, as the vertebrates began to occupy new niche environments, the abilities of species and the brain regions that supported them were becoming shaped by different demands. New habitats, prey and predators favoured processing senses and actions in different ways. Some changes

The evolving vertebrate brain

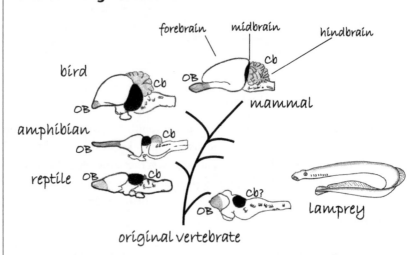

The original vertebrate evolved into all the major classes we know today, with the jawless lamprey fish thought to be its closest living relative. The "tripartite" ground plan of the brain has been preserved, with modifications reflecting the demands of different evolutionary "niches". For example, the size of the olfactory bulb in some mammals (marked OB) reflects greater dependence on smell. Differences in the extent of cerebellum circuitry (marked Cb) appear meant bigger brains but the brain, more than most organs, is expensive to run.[70] Over time, extra brain power has only evolved when its value for survival could justify the additional energy it consumed. Brain tissue that failed this test diminished over time, causing some brain regions in some species to grow smaller.

And so, as vertebrates begun to occupy different niches, they diverged from our common vertebrate ancestor through the processes of natural selection. The brains and learning abilities of today's vertebrates display some important differences but still retain some underlying similarities too. We see a relative difference in the proportion of brain regions – but still the same basic ground plan. We see relative differences in abilities – but still the same set of basic learning systems.

Some of the regions used by these learning systems exist under the cortex – the so-called "sub-cortical" regions. They include the thalamus, through which most of our senses enter the brain, and the striatum – an important structure involved with motivation and processing reward. Structures that are heavily involved with memory formation include the hippocampus and,

related to everyday demands for movement coordination, particularly those involving manipulation of the environment (e.g. nest building).

The human forebrain has expanded to hide the midbrain, but the section view below reveals the same basic plan as other vertebrates. As in the evolutionary tree just encountered, the olfactory bulb and cerebellum are in grey, and the midbrain is in black. The small olfactory bulb reflects our diminished reliance on smell compared with other mammals.

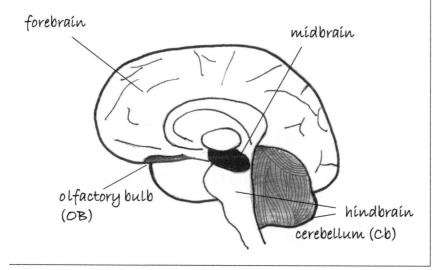

particularly when emotional content is involved, the amygdala. Since this book is the story of our own learning brain, these sub-cortical structures are drawn here in human form. And explanations of learning processes in this chapter will also often be in human terms – even though it's another couple of million years until we arrive. But . . . this could be viewed as just a shameless bias towards our own species, since our common ancestry means other vertebrates have versions of these regions and processes too.

If the human cortex was made of glass, these sub-cortical structures on one side of the brain would look something like this:

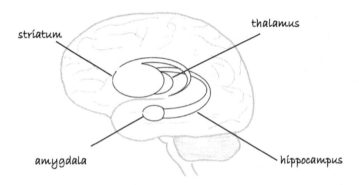

These structures are also mirrored on the other side, so we have a left and a right amygdala, a left and right hippocampus etc.

To illustrate the different learning systems, think about an expedition to collect shells on a beach. Thanks to supermarkets, most of us don't forage for shellfish to eat anymore, but it's just the type of gathering exercise that would once have been critical for our survival. A successful expedition can depend on the same set of learning systems possessed by many other hungry vertebrates. However, before any of the four learning systems can kick in and help, information about the outside world needs to find its way in through our senses to our brain.

Brain inputs to four learning systems: the thalamus and olfactory bulb

Learning in the beach scenario will rely heavily on sensory input: the different patterns of the shells, their texture and the sound of your friends when they discover something or warn you the tide is coming in. In all vertebrates, the *thalamus*ᶦ is the gateway to the cortex for all the information coming in from seeing, touching and hearing, as well as for sensory information of what's going on in your digestive system – such as the signs of hunger. In our glass brain, the thalamus is peeking out (and shown in black) from deep within:

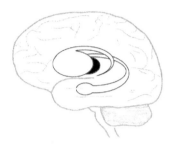

The thalamus is much larger in amniotes (animals that don't lay eggs in water). It's particularly large in mammals and birds, where it's divided up into many densely packed parcels of neurons related to different senses, movements and emotions.[71] Unlike the cerebral cortex, we know very little about how it functions across different species.[72] What we do know suggests that, as species have specialized in different inputs, so this has become reflected in the structure of the thalamus and how it's connected with the cortex.[73]

The one sense that does not enter the cortex through the thalamus is olfaction (or smell). In vertebrates, this goes directly into the cortex, entering at the olfactory bulb. Different species vary in how much they navigate using smell, and the size of their bulb varies accordingly.[74] Generally, humans don't use smell in a very sophisticated way and we have a relatively small bulb. We don't tend to find our way with smell or, apart from the occasional perfume, use it to communicate with. Smell will not be that useful for collecting shells either. However, for early and many modern mammals, it may have been so critical for survival that it drove initial increases in the size of mammalian cortex. The changing shape of the brain, based on fossil skull cavities, also tells us that the sense of touch was improving amongst early mammals.[75] These additional sensory skills would have helped survival, particularly when providing parental care. Smell and touch offer greater communication and sensitivity, and so they can help ensure infants get the warmth and attention they need. Greater sensitivity to touch through facial hair (whiskers) would also have helped early mammals to navigate in the dark underground where they sheltered. All these extra-sensory needs drove the evolution of the mammalian thalamus in a slightly different, more complex direction.[76]

The grand library of the brain: the cerebral cortex and the organisation of information

As you scan the different shells, even if you have never seen them before and know nothing about shore life, you will be learning to categorise them. These categories help you identify which are different or potentially valuable. The amazing thing about this categorisation is that you can do it without any feedback. No-one and nothing is telling you when you make a mistake – and yet somehow you can just work this out, and the more you categorise the better you get at it. This type of learning relies on the neural networks that exist in your cortex – the largest and wrinkliest part of your forebrain:

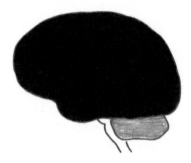

It may seem odd that we can learn without feedback, but think about a trainee librarian. Left unsupervised in a room of new stock, the trainee can still sort the books according to some basic similarities in their content, despite not knowing the official filing system. When the supervisor arrives back, he/she might make a few changes, but the trainee's work means the library is already a little more organised and useful for finding an individual book.

Like the trainee, the cerebral cortex is also good at building links based on similarities and differences. It can automatically make associations and so link together similar inputs. It can organise information in a way that makes it more useful for future purposes – even when it's not clear what these purposes will be. Unsupervised learning helps us pick out patterns emerging through the vast and noisy flow of data reaching us from the outside world.[77] It allows information (and particularly the bits for describing the world in terms of similarities and differences) to be efficiently filed, ready for reactivation by some relevant event. This ordering and linking of new information with old is an important part of how we make meaning.

All vertebrates have a structure that could be called a cortex[ii] but its shape and size varies across species. Mammals and birds have developed larger brains in relation to their body mass than amphibians and reptiles,[78] and this is due largely to the size of their forebrain. Based on living examples and fossil evidence from casts of skulls, this expansion of the forebrain (so-called *encephalisation*) occurred gradually over time and happened independently in mammals and birds. This is an example of how evolution sometimes causes convergence rather than divergence – resulting in a similar feature shared by two, quite distant, species. Birds display some impressive mental abilities that may be related to the expanded size of their forebrain.

Another difference between the brain of mammals and other animals can be seen in the layering of their cortex. The mammalian cortex has a six-layered (or "laminar") structure consisting of many different types of neurons.[79–82] In birds the structure resembles that of slabs rather than layers, and reptiles have a three-layered arrangement. Scientists are still trying work out what a multi-layered cortex means for our mental abilities, but it's thought the six-layered structure helps us attend to vital features and filter out unwanted information, as well as supporting our unsupervised learning.[83]

Unsupervised learning processes are largely unconscious, but sometimes you need to pay conscious attention to information for a few moments and the cortex plays an important role here too. Suppose you remember finding some particularly nice shells last week, and want to know which direction might lead you to them again. You need to recall and focus on the features of where you were that day and, at the same time, consciously compare them in "your mind's eye" with what you see in front of you now. This ability to consciously attend to information is referred to as your *working memory* capacity and it's limited. It's thought humans can only hold about seven pieces of information in our heads at once.[84] When we use our working memory, the neurons that represent a piece of information persist in their firing. Brain imaging has revealed this sustained activity occurs particularly in the frontal regions of our cortex, as we try to simultaneously represent and process several ideas at once.[85] Working memory is of great interest to educators. When we first learn something, we tend to hold a lot of the new information in our consciousness when applying it. This creates a bottleneck that makes it difficult to learn more until using this information has become a more automatic and unconscious process. For that reason, our working memory capacity strongly predicts our ability to move forward with our learning, and so also our academic and professional success.

Fine tuning movement: the cerebellum

Sometimes you get some very obvious feedback on your performance – such as when you try some difficult manoeuvre and end up falling over. Balancing on rocks while holding your collection of shells can be particularly tricky – but, by being sensitive to how you are balancing (or, more accurately, how you might not be), you can learn to get the hang of it. The cerebellum is key to this error-based type of learning involving our fine movements. The cerebellum is part of the hindbrain and can be seen protruding at the back of the cortex:

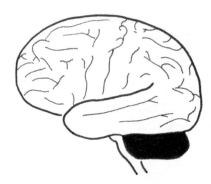

We used to think the cerebellum was just about controlling movement, rather than learning. For example, the cerebellum of amphibians is smaller than other vertebrates, and that may be because less care is required when moving closer to the ground. However, it now appears the cerebellum has a more important role in how we develop our view of the world.[86] For one thing, it helps you link the movement information your brain outputs with the incoming sensory information about where your body is and how it's moving.[87] How well your movement turns out (an external error signal) helps you adjust the way these two sets of information are connected. In this way, the cerebellum helps tune your brain's representation of your body (e.g. your posture) and of the world (e.g. the rocks), and to learn how these two things are connected. This is sometimes called supervised learning, as if a supervisor was providing clear training and feedback about how well you're doing ("you're closer, close – perfect!"). Neural networks use this feedback to organise themselves and relate sensory input to motor output.[88] The cerebellum is one of the least understood regions of the brain, but it helps us build a model in our cortex of our world and ourselves. In this way, it contributes to a wide range of abilities less obviously related to movement, including rhythm and language.[89]

Moving for advantage: the basal ganglia and reinforcement learning system

As you move off the rocks and start scanning the sandy beach for shells, you're no longer having to focus on putting one foot in front of the other.

Walking is one of those many things we can do automatically without thinking – like chewing and moving our eyes. To do these things, we turn stored programmes of movement into actions. To avoid walking accidentally into the sea and getting our feet wet, we must apply these programmes in a controlled way that ensures the best outcomes.

The basal ganglia are a system of structures across the hindbrain and midbrain that has evolved for this type of movement control. They work in an essentially similar way across all vertebrates, and it appears we inherited this system from the first (jawless) fishes. The modern lamprey belongs to the oldest surviving class of vertebrates[90] and, like ancient fish, is also jawless. In the lamprey, we see a basal ganglia system conserved in vertebrates across deep time – around half a billion years.[91] The striatum is involved with our response to many pleasures, such as food, but this is also the main input to the basal ganglia:

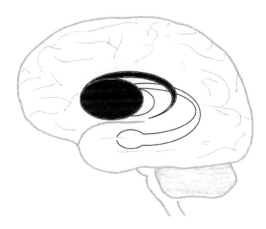

The striatum is stimulated by what's happening in the cortex but also by neurons from the midbrain. These neurons have chemical synapses that use the neurotransmitter dopamine, and they activate in response to reward and its anticipation. This response in the striatum is key to producing the best actions for reaping these rewards, such as when a frog must generate the best movement of its tongue for catching a fly.

To achieve this, two types of pathway from the striatum influence the basal ganglia to send "Go" and "No-Go" messages to centres in the midbrain and hindbrain that issue the movement commands. Via the thalamus, output from the striatum also changes how these movements are represented in the cortex. In this way, the basal ganglia orchestrate the coordination of individual actions required for behaviours like moving and feeding.

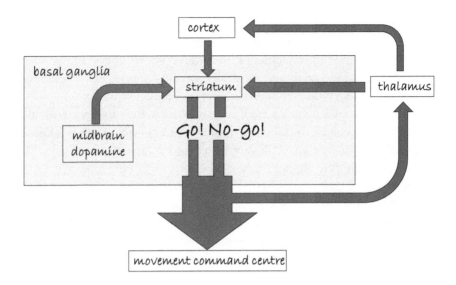

For most of these everyday repetitive movements, most of what the basal ganglia needs as input is the sensory and other information arriving through the thalamus. Very little, if any, input is needed from the cortex.[92] In amphibians, for example, the input gets relayed almost directly from the thalamus to the striatum,[93] with little chance of being modified by the cortex.

However, for many species, the survival advantages of learning to select different actions rapidly in a changing world were becoming greater on land. This learning is potentially more complex than catching a fly. Finding enough food could mean foraging in environments where the returns from different sources were constantly changing – and that presented a challenge. It meant an animal must keep updating the potential value of multiple changing options, exploiting those currently more rewarding, but also occasionally exploring the others. In this scenario, short-term outcomes must not be allowed to eclipse longer-term benefits. That means a policy is needed to inform decisions and that policy must be constantly updated. Even mathematicians have struggled to find a straightforward solution to this problem. It's a challenge that has been studied for decades by experts in artificial intelligence and statistics.

One set of solutions – with a biological basis – comes under the heading of *reinforcement learning*. In this type of learning, important information about the situation is represented flexibly in the cortex, supporting the calculation of a "prediction error" after every action. This is a different type of error from just being told that a movement was correct or incorrect. In this type of learning, the prediction error is the difference between the anticipated and observed outcome – with a higher prediction error implying a happy surprise and a greater likelihood the action will be repeated. This is coded by the size of dopamine release from the midbrain into those regions of the striatum involved with selecting that action. When that's done, the striatum helps to reorganise the representation of the whole situation in the cortex. These processes are thought to be the basis of how rodents[94] and birds[95] forage for food, learning about what's paying off as they go. Neuroimaging studies have shown how this dopamine signal informs human foraging too,[96] and helps us make some economic decisions. For example, when people were searching a virtual maze for sums of money, researchers could observe connectivity strengthening between regions of the cortex representing the value of particular routes and those parts of the striatum that were helping to make the decisions.[97]

The advantages of such efficient foraging favoured the increasing involvement of the cortex. Along the evolutionary road that leads to the human species, the cortex has generally become more interconnected with the basal ganglia. There appear to be dramatic increases in such connections at key moments in the evolutionary story, such as when the egg-laying animals (amniotes) arrived and when the mammals appeared.

Making memories: the hippocampus and declarative memory system

As you stroll along the beach, you might remember a place where yesterday you found some particularly good shells, causing you to immediately change course and forage there instead. But how did the memory of what happened yesterday get "stored" in your brain so clearly that it could get pulled out like that and placed in your consciousness (i.e. in your working memory)?

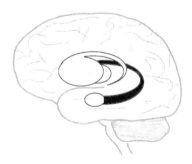

Making a memory for what's happened in the past is a very useful learning ability and, at least for humans, we call it declarative memory formation (because we can make it conscious and declare it). The hippocampus is the brain region most famously involved with making this type of long-term memory. The hippocampus helps us to record a specific new event but also to link the new experience with previous ones based on common features. It appears central to the process of recording a long-term memory in the cortex of "what" the experience was all generally about, tied up with the "when" of its happening.

In evolutionary terms, the adaptive advantage of this system is clear. Survival can routinely rely on remembering what happened in a place, and what sort of food or danger you've generally encountered there. A strong ability to remember the "where" appears to have been conserved in the vertebrate brain, judging by closer relatives of our common ancestor – the fish. Goldfish, for example, appear to form mental maps of the areas they inhabit.[98] On the other hand, a goldfish's memory of what happened in these areas seems much weaker. Possibly the hippocampus was initially limited to processing spatial information and, amongst fish and amphibians, remains so. The arrival of our true "what-where" capacity appeared to come after the arrival of amphibians and fishes, but before mammals and reptiles diverged.[99]

When memory for an event is first represented in the brain, it is fragile and vulnerable to being lost. Studies with humans and rodents suggest that sleep helps make our memories more permanent. Sleep is a generally neglected issue amongst educators, but it's necessary precisely because we must learn so much in a day. It has been called "the price we pay for plasticity"[100] – and organisms without a central nervous system just don't seem to need it. In mammals that are awake, combined information about an event is first *encoded* (or represented) as neural activity in the hippocampus during wakeful experience but, during sleeping, these fresh representations are reactivated and reorganised in a process known as *consolidation*. They are then *stored* as longer-lasting memories in the cortex. So, although we may not be consciously aware of passing from one stage to the next, there are three basic brain processes involved with forming a memory:

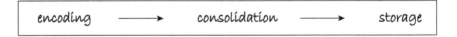

encoding ⟶ consolidation ⟶ storage

This is illustrated most strikingly by human neuroimaging studies. One of these reveals how the sleeping brain reproduces similar neural activities to those activated by whatever we were doing when we were awake.[101] This reactivation of fresh memories is thought to happen during deep sleep, when the brain produces slow waves (less than one per second) of synchronised electrical brain activity. The consolidation provided by slow-wave sleep can improve memory of the context, but it also helps generalise and extract the gist of the memory. In this way, sleep helps us store and later recall the memory in a form that's more ready to be used in new situations, with the unhelpful detail edited out. The importance of sleep for learning has also been demonstrated by educational researchers (see box below).

Teens and computer games: when the "price for plasticity" doesn't get paid . . .

The relationship of brain plasticity to sleep has some educational implications, particularly in the digital world. For example, our sleep can often get disrupted by our use of technology, particularly if it is a very arousing activity. The enthusiasm of teenagers for playing computer games has raised concerns about how this may be impacting on their sleep[102] and, consequently, their learning. In one study, a group of young teenagers were asked to vary their use of technology before immediately doing a "pseudo" homework task that involved memorising facts.[103] On one occasion they experienced no technology, on another they watched television between 6 and 7 pm, and on another they played computer games instead during this period. When computer games were played, the greatest loss of slow-wave sleep occurred. This is the type of sleep thought to be most important for consolidating declarative memory, and children's memory for their "homework" was also least on days that followed this activity.

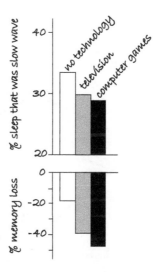

A comparison across animals helps provide some clues about how sleep evolved alongside learning ability. Birds sleep in a rather fragmented way (periods of 1–4 minutes, often with one eye open) but, like mammals, they experience slow-wave sleep and their learning suffers if sleep gets disrupted. For example, chicks can quickly learn to follow whatever object they first come across after birth (usually their mother). This is called "imprinting", but it appears critical for the chick to experience sleep within around 9 hours of the imprinting training, if the memory is to be lasting.[104] Less is known about the sleep of reptiles and amphibians, so it's difficult to know whether all vertebrates experience slow-wave sleep. However, in the last two decades, experiments with insects suggest the basic system (i.e. reactivating and reorganising information) may have been conserved since before vertebrates appeared.[105] Insects don't experience slow-wave sleep, but bees show better memory for new routes home to their hive after a nap.[106] When experience shapes the neural connections of fruit-fly, these connections then get reshaped by sleep.[100,107] It's not easy measuring learning in a fruit-fly but some crafty experimenters have done so based on unrequited love. Unsuccessful mating can be arranged for male fruit-flies by placing them for a few hours with other males laced with female pheromones. After many frustrated attempts to mate, a hapless male learns not to be fooled by flies that only smell like females. This learning – as you may already have guessed – is helped by a little sleep. A sleeping fruit-fly even shows reduced firing in its neurons,[108] which is a key feature of the sleep state that has also be found in worms.[109,110] Sleep and learning have evolved over deep time:[109]

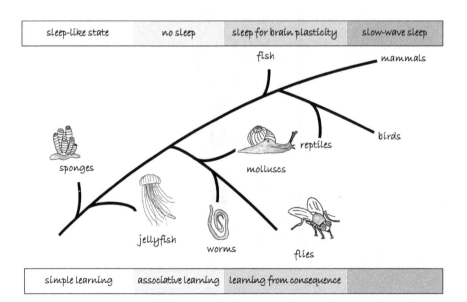

Emotion can be an important part of a memory. Suppose, when collecting your shells, you wander into a cave where once you were almost trapped by an incoming tide. Or you might encounter a dangerous area of quicksand or poisonous jellyfish you've come across before. These past adventures would have stirred some strong feelings at the time and, as a result, the memory of the event and its emotion come back to warn you away. This seems a particularly important type of learning for survival, so how does the vertebrate brain mark these emotional memories as "special"?

The amygdala is a primary structure for the experiencing and processing of emotions. It's also a key region for emotional learning and well connected with the hippocampus, which is its neighbouring structure:

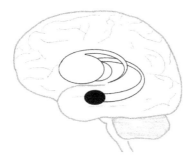

This coupling of the amygdala (emotion) and hippocampus (memory) allows for the efficient emotional tagging of memories. During an emotionally arousing event, activation of the amygdala marks the experience as important and enhances plasticity in the hippocampus and other brain regions, so making the experience more memorable. Across vertebrates we see primitive examples of how emotion can improve memory and these include fear associations.[111,112] Even the much-maligned goldfish – sometimes unfairly ridiculed for its memory – can manage to avoid something previously associated with danger.[113-115]

However, many animals who lay eggs on land, such as reptiles, birds and mammals, are capable of more sophisticated emotional learning and "new" regions of the amygdala have evolved in these creatures.[116] This may reflect the additional demands of protecting vulnerable eggs and young. Only mammals, for example, can learn by frustration and change their behaviour when they've missed out on an anticipated reward.[111,117] Mammals also appear to have evolved a response to a mildly stressful situation that can increase our ability to learn from it (see box overleaf).

Is mild stress good or bad for learning?

Studies with humans and rodents suggest that stress triggers hormones (glucocorticoids and noradrenaline) that influence how the amygdala functions and this, in turn, can positively impact on encoding processes in other regions of the brain, including the hippocampus.[118] This helps explain how *mild* stress has been associated with improved human learning in some educational experiences.[119,120] Lingering glucocorticoids can further help this process by reducing the effect of new, and therefore irrelevant, information during consolidation of the new memory. On the other hand, if the stress occurs a while before the learning, these lingering hormones can reduce the processing and encoding of its memory.[121] So, depending on timing, mild stress can produce opposite effects on learning:[122]

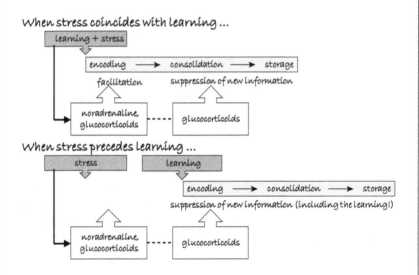

Stress can also make it more difficult to retrieve a memory later and apply it to a new problem.[123] Individuals who are anxious about mathematics, for example, under-perform in tests due to the stress they experience during the test. This is due to reduced working memory[124] rather than a lack of knowledge and understanding. Note that mild stress should not be confused with the life-changing effects of the extraordinary and severe stress that some children must suffer, often due to deprivation or maltreatment. In many such cases, this can result in long-term damage to the stress response,[125] lasting alterations in the structure and function of the brain[126] and problems in emotional responding that continue into later life.

Learning systems are interconnected

At any particular moment in our trip to the seaside, one learning system appears to have been more useful than the others. Vertebrates do not, however, have to switch off one system before turning on another. Instead, two, three or all their learning systems can be used together. Even the simplest of learning situations will probably need more than one system and these systems have evolved to interact in most everyday learning tasks. We've already talked about the cerebellum and cerebral cortex working together in supervised learning, and how the basal ganglia and cortex work together in reinforcement learning. The cerebellum and the basal ganglia are also interconnected, so that the output of the cerebellum influences the input of the basal ganglia and vice-versa.[127] The interconnected nature of these four learning systems has some implications for education. For instance, the uptake of midbrain dopamine that guides foraging can also improve memory formation.[128] That interaction may have evolved to make the location of a rich food source more memorable for vertebrates, but it can also predict when humans learn educational facts in a learning-game (see box overleaf).

Jurassic life meets Armageddon

About 65.5 Myr, the reign of the dinosaurs came to a sudden end when an asteroid collided with the Earth, creating what is now the Chicxulub crater in Mexico. Debris from the crater soared upward into the atmosphere and halfway to the moon before raining back upon our planet. Within three days, this lethal fall of burning rock had ignited raging wildfires from North America to India. Dust from the impact combined with the smoke from the fires to choke the skies. The Earth was plunged into a "nuclear winter", with plants dying from lack of sunlight and food chains collapsing.

The details of the ensuing death and destruction are still the subject of argument, but versions include incineration, suffocation and starvation in varying proportions. The global extent of the devastation is more undisputable. No large, non-marine reptile, bird or mammal survived or, in other words, no vertebrate that was unable to hide underground, in tree cavities or underwater.

Mammals had evolved several features that may have contributed to their survival during this terrible time. Firstly, an ability to hibernate would have helped them to remain in a subterranean refuge for a longer period than other animals, escaping the short- and medium-term effects of the asteroid strike.[129,130] Secondly, by the beginning of the Jurassic, mammals had evolved larger nasal cavities and olfactory bulbs, and their cortex had doubled in size.[75]

Our learning system for sourcing food can influence our memory for information

Researchers devised an educational game where adults foraged for points in four boxes, but could only keep the points if they could correctly answer the question that followed.[131]

When participants guessed incorrectly, they were told the correct answer and, since questions repeated, pretty soon they began to learn these answers. Whether participants could recall the correct answer did not seem to depend on the stakes available (i.e. the points in the box). Instead, it depended on an estimate of midbrain dopamine (based on prediction error – or how much more was in the box than the participant had expected):

Pick a box ...

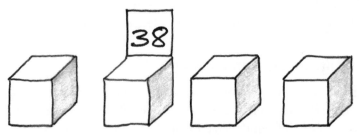

To win these points, which of these is an alkali metal?

Mercury   Sodium   Copper   Iron

The exact mechanisms are not well understood, but other studies have made this link between midbrain dopamine and memory formation.[132] This link may provide a fresh perspective on the use of reward to incentivise learning, since we know midbrain dopamine is influenced by many things, including the recent history of receiving rewards[133] and, in humans at least, the context of the reward[134] and the presence of peers.[135] It also appears that primates, including ourselves, generate a greater midbrain dopamine response when the anticipated rewards are uncertain – i.e. when there is a strong element of chance.[136] This idea has spawned some successful interventions that have improved educational learning through offering rewards that rely on a bit of luck, such as throwing dice or spinning a wheel of fortune.[137,138]

Before the cataclysm struck, enhanced equipment for identifying and processing smells would have been helpful in a world of dangerous and enticing
scents and odours, but the cortex is also helpful for learning associations. It
is very plastic and, in abnormal circumstances such as trauma, cortex usually used for one sense can begin to be employed for learning associations
of another type. Perhaps the flexibility provided by this additional cortex,
although initially evolved for a Jurassic lifestyle, may have helped early
mammals flourish in their new habitats? If so, this would not be the last time
that a mammal would benefit from being able, without genetic change, to
"recycle" its cortex to help fit a new environment (see Chapters 7 and 8).

Mammals, of course, were not the only big group of survivors. Birds,
or at least some of those able to feed from the waters or burrow like kiwis,
also survived.[139] However, 75% or more of all species were extinguished.[140]
Following the disaster, the remaining vertebrates emerged from their hid-
ing places into a world that was somewhat empty. The old order was gone
and survival would mean exploiting new food chains and adapting to new
ecological zones.[141] After the meteor strike, the evolution of all surviving
groups of vertebrates exploded.

Notes

i Dorsal thalamus.
ii More strictly referred to as the "pallium" in non-mammal vertebrates.

4

THE SOCIAL PRIMATE

AFTER THE NUCLEAR WINTER of the extinction event, the surviving mammals found themselves in a world that would, over the next 10 million years, get slowly warmer. We cannot be sure of the exact causes for this global warming[142] but the changes in CO_2 levels suggest massive injections of carbon into the atmosphere from volcanic activity, possibly bolstered by warm seas releasing their stored gas.[143] Whatever was behind it, we know by 55 Myr there were widespread tropical and subtropical conditions.

From as early as **65 Myr**, alongside this warming, mammals began to emerge with distinct primate features.[144] The early primates were rather small, nocturnal and lived chiefly on insects. Their brains were also small – suggesting mental abilities similar to the mammals around them. They would have had their own share of familiar learning systems for organising information, for foraging, for adjusting their movements and for recalling events from the past. Some features of their skulls, however, suggest this new animal had found a novel evolutionary niche – a new way of fitting into the environment.

The fossilised skulls of early primates provide several tantalising clues about what this different "way of living" might have been. For over a century, the dominant story of how primates evolved was the "arboreal hypothesis": it was simply the move to a tree-dwelling life that drove change. However, many other animals live in trees (for example, tree shrews) and their brains and skulls are not like a primate's. We can see from the primate skull that their eyes, unlike other mammals, were beginning to converge. Moreover, the skull cavity shows that the size of the brain was not just increasing, but its shape was also changing. The issue of a brain's shape is important because different parts of a primate brain are associated with different functions (see box opposite). Why, as well as a general increase in size, were regions associated with vision expanding, while the olfactory bulb (for smell) was shrinking?[145]

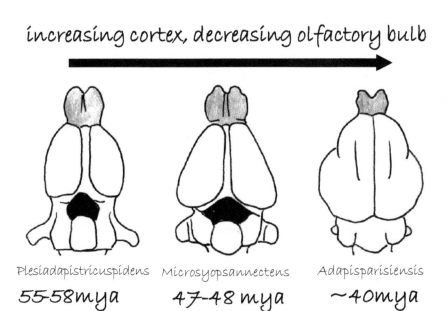

increasing cortex, decreasing olfactory bulb

Plesiadapistricuspidens — 55-58mya

Microsyopsannectens — 47-48 mya

Adapisparisiensis — ~40mya

The answer appears to be a change in how food was being collected. Primates have the grasping hands and feet required for foraging at the ends of branches.[146] This arrangement allows the hind limbs to suspend their bodies while their forelimbs tackle the food, as in these hanging lemurs:

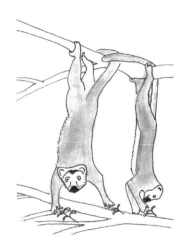

Apart from a few primate-like marsupials and some flying animals, primates are the only major group of vertebrates that routinely perform this feat. Doing tricky things while hanging off a branch may be the act that initially defined the primate. Having adopted this way of feeding, food on faraway branches could be reached – provided it could be spotted. Early primates were predators and the food was most likely to be a moving target of insects. Convergent eyes, like those of cats and hawks, were also now more advantageous, because they could help penetrate the cluttered forest for prey and allow the fine judging of distance when closing in.[147] In 2002, a 56-Myr precursor to fully modern primates was found in Wyoming with potential grasping abilities but with no convergent forward-facing eyes. This does appear to confirm that primates evolved their branch-hanging antics first and their converging eyes came later.

From these early primates evolved today's lemurs and tarsiers (small insect-eating nocturnal predators with large eyes), but also the lineage of

---

The lobes of the primate cortex – and what they do

No single brain region is entirely dedicated to any one type of everyday activity. We do not, for example, have a bit of our brain that is exclusively for maths, creativity or music. But the basic underlying mental abilities (or cognitive functions) needed for these activities are associated more with some regions than others. Moreover, there is a mapping of basic function to different regions that is broadly similar across primates. For example, the frontal lobes are essential for regulating emotion and behaviour, and they have a key role in supporting conscious reasoning and working memory. The temporal lobes are those cortical regions most involved with long-term memory, including visual memory, as well as the processing of sound. The parietal lobes are heavily involved in connecting together information from our different senses, and the occipital lobes are critical for vision:

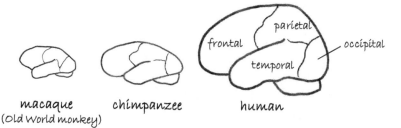

macaque (Old World monkey) chimpanzee human

Any everyday task, however, calls on these functions in different ways. A particular task will prompt a large and broadly distributed set of networks across these lobes to communicate with each other in a way that is specific to that task.

"anthropoid monkeys". The great apes – the family of animals to which we belong – would one day evolve from these anthropoids. Unlike their predecessors, the anthropoids were visual predators who hunted by day, evolving larger bodies and more diversified diets that included fruit and leaves. This change in diet may have helped drive some of the new changes we see in the proportions of the anthropoid brain. Modern primates harvest leaves and fruit in a certain way: by visually guiding and controlling their arm to reach for the fruit, and manipulating their hand to "preshape" it just before grasping. Greater control makes this complex manoeuvre much more effective. This would have favoured the types of increase we see in the occipital and temporal lobes of the brain for processing visual information, and in parietal regions for connecting the visual information to movement information in the frontal lobes.[148–150]

The clearest examples of early great apes have been found in Germany and Turkey and date from around 16 Myr. Based on this fossil evidence, these larger primates had thickly enamelled teeth and a robust jaw for munching vegetation. They had a more powerful grasp for moving around above and below branch level[151] and were also now tailless – the feature commonly used to tell apes and monkeys apart. This suggests they were moving around the trees with a slower, grasping approach without needing the balance and leaping skills that a tail can provide.[152] So many key events in our primate history have occurred in Africa, you might assume apes started here too. However, evidence such as German and Turkish fossils suggest the origins of apes in Eurasia,[153] in which case an "into Africa" migration of the common ancestor of all living African apes happened sometime after

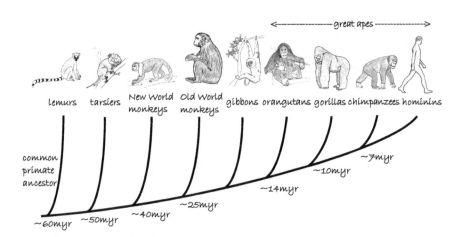

10 Myr.[154] Wherever they began, it was in Africa (around **7 Myr**) that we find one line of these apes diverging. One branch led to bonobos and chimpanzees (our closest genetic non-human relative) and another to a group of bipedal primates known as the hominins, which would later include archaic and eventually modern humans.[155]

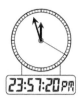

The social brain hypothesis

From early on, we find a general trend of expansion in the primate brain. This was an expensive trend. Per kilogram, the cost of maintaining the brain is 8–10 times higher than the muscles in your arms and legs. Therefore, more brain means a lot more food is needed – and a greater risk of starvation if food stocks run low. So there had to be a good reason *why* primates would benefit from having a bigger brain than most other mammals. Beyond the initial tree-hanging routine, the reason appears to be the increasingly social nature of their niche.

Primates are intensely social creatures and they live together in groups ranging up to 800 in size.[156] As with the joining together of cells into multicellular forms, being part of a bunch offers some obvious protection. The initial impetus for this increase in sociality may have been saying goodbye to the nightlife, since daytime living makes the sharing of protection and warnings much more important. As well as reducing the chances of getting eaten,[157] communal life increases the chances of finding and defending food[158] and can even help repel attacks by members of your own species.[158] Of course, as most of us know, group living does present challenges. For one thing, being with others who share your tastes in food means potential competition – either one of your peers may grab and eat everything you find, or they may gobble their own discoveries before you arrive for your share. Amongst primates, what that share might be is usually determined competitively. Living in a group, therefore, ends up being a skilled mixture of collaboration and competition – and a need to change tactics depending on who you're dealing with. "Understandings", in terms of bonds and conflicts between individuals, help prevent constant conflict by sorting things out in a non-lethal manner. These social relations minimise short-term losses from arguments in everyday business, while protecting the long-term gain of working as a group. What makes this really challenging, however, is that the world is always changing, and so these social contracts have to change too. For example, as food gets scarcer, a group of chimpanzees will forage more widely and have further to travel home. But if food gets so scarce that the commute no longer justifies the pay off, it makes sense for the large group to split into smaller new groupings. New groupings mean new interactions and new contracts.

Inevitably, then, surviving through flexible social behaviour means that things get messy and complicated and primates need sophisticated tactics for coping. Unlike many other animals, primates develop complex one-to-one relations with each other that are not just for reproduction (e.g. they also happen between same-sex individuals). They invest considerable time and energy in maintaining and building their social standing in groups that are only semi-permanent. The larger the group, the more complex things get. Rapid learning is required to discriminate between individuals in the group, to maintain a tally of groomings received, to record how past favours have influenced returns, etc. When the group reaches a certain size, the amount of mental processing required to deal with all this becomes very challenging. This predicts that every primate species, including our own, has an optimal social group size, which is basically as big as their brain can cope with. More specifically, large groups test the ability of our cortex to organise information, so we find a relationship between its relative size in different primate species and their average group size – i.e. the social complexity of their world:[159]

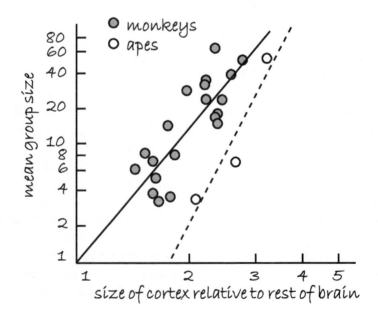

In the modern age, many of us use social network sites to maintain contact with very large groups. The effect these efforts have on our plastic cortex demonstrates the challenging nature of this task. Moreover, the general success of our species in maintaining intimacy using face-to-face or virtual networks is still predicted, as for other primates, by the size of our cortex (see box below).

Human social networks – and your brain on Facebook

By looking at the relationship between group size and cortex size in non-human primates, the upper limit on a human network has been predicted to be around 150.[160] Later studies confirmed this figure for our everyday social networks.[161,162] The limitations on social network size are illustrated in social terms by diminishing intimacy as size increases. Studies of Facebook behaviour show online networks mirror offline ones, with a similar limit upon the number of online friends we can include in a functioning social group.[163]

Our primate sociality also shapes our brain during our lifetime, and a relationship exists between an individual's online social network and their brain structure. In a study of adults, it was shown that the number of friends declared online predicted the size of cortical regions associated with social perception and associative memory.[164] The direction of cause and effect is not known – either the physical dimensions of our brain limit our Facebook network or, more likely, the structure of our plastic cortex changes, over time, in response to our Facebook demands. Either way, this study shows the extent to which our cortical capacities are still closely entwined with our complex social lives.

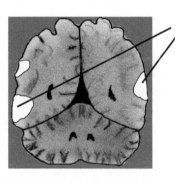

Regions coloured white vary in their size according to number of friends on social networks (e.g. Facebook).

(This view is as if the brain was sliced along the dotted line.)

The primate neuronal-packing advantage

Evolved increases in brain size were much more significant for primates because each time the primate brain expanded, it did so in a way that resulted in many more neurons than if it were any other species. Earlier in evolution, mammals diverged in apparently small ways in terms of how their neurons multiplied during development and what volume they occupied. Exactly how this works is still unclear, but it resulted in species having different "scaling rules" for the number of neurons gained for the same genetic increase in brain size.[165,166] Early primates must have evolved particularly impressive ways to pack in their neurons – a genetic feature that would have huge significance for their descendants, including us. For example, if evolution resulted in a rat with a 10-fold increase in its neurons, this would mean a 35-fold larger brain. In contrast, a primate can evolve a 10-fold increase in neurons by having a brain only 10 times as large.[167]

Primates are interested in others' business

Of course, the advantage of a larger brain wasn't all about one-to-one interactions within the group.[168] There are many other ways in which social brain power can improve survival. It can help strategise during conflict between groups, meet the mental demands of foraging in a greater space[169] and help cope with the complications of infant-care during these foraging sessions.[170]

However, probably the most obvious talent that distinguishes primates from other animals is their interest and ability to understand *events they are not directly involved in*. In other words, primates are great at eavesdropping. By the time primates had lost most of their olfactory bulb, they were on their way to becoming experts in nosing around the social world instead, getting stuck into the business of friends and enemies that was not directly their own. This social nosiness is an important skill for making daily decisions when competing and collaborating for patchy resources. A single individual in a group is always at risk of being dominated by others around them and successful strategies are more than just about standing ground. Typically, you need cooperation with allies against opponents, which makes it crucial to attend to and understand the social ups and downs of those around you.

More than other mammals, primates track the relationships between others and act on the information they receive. For example, following an aggressive incident between chimpanzees, uninvolved bystanders will often approach one of the opponents and take sides with them by offering affiliation. Sometimes it is the aggressor that receives the support, but more often it is the victim. Bonobos, a type of chimpanzee, have been observed approaching those who have suffered conflict, sometimes offering consolation with touching and embracing.[171] This is more likely to happen when the victims are closely-bonded partners or relations. A systematic and broad social awareness is also seen in the behaviour of adolescent chimpanzees, as they first establish their position in the hierarchy. Their tactics reveal they already have a good understanding of the ranking. They begin by threatening low-ranking females, then move onto higher-ranking ones. Then they begin to work their way from the bottom upwards through the male hierarchy.[172] Following a conflict, relations of an aggressor are more likely to be attacked later by those of the victim, even though none of these individuals were actively involved in the original aggression. After reconciliation between a victim and an aggressor, increased levels of post-conflict affiliation between their relations have also been observed. All this shows they have been paying close attention to social goings-on that they have not directly been involved with. Primates can also keep a log of others' familial relations. Many mammals will recognise the sound of their own offspring but when a female vervet monkey hears a call from an infant that's not hers, she will look towards the mother.[173]

The social awareness of primates is impressive. They anticipate and plan how to form temporary coalitions and long-term alliances, remember the outcomes of these ventures and learn from them. Although some animals, such as ravens,[174] also show an awareness of hierarchy, primates excel in the efficiency and variety of the social strategies they employ – particularly when it comes to third parties. For example, chimpanzee males compete for powerful partners using diverse coalitionary tactics that one might call political.[175,176] These include performing "separating interventions" that keep apart rivals, and they will support others to confront those who have formed coalitions against them.[176–178] Some of this sophistication certainly does appear to depend on brain size,[179] because smaller primates more often employ simpler strategies such as the "gang-attack" coalitions of rhesus macaque males.[180]

The primate theory of mind

The political cunning of primates suggests they can learn about each other's emotional state and predict their behaviour. So . . . did primates, before humans, already have the ability to consider the beliefs, intentions and perspectives of others? In other words, do primates have a theory of mind? This has been a controversial question, chiefly because of our tendency to assume our mental abilities are unique to humans. Data has been published on both sides of the argument, and it has been difficult for non-experts to know what they should conclude. The best scientists always base their views on the evidence and, since evidence collects and understanding develops, they must be allowed to change their views accordingly. These changes, however, often represent significant milestones in the debate. In 1997, two of the foremost experts on primate cognition, Michael Tomasello and Josep Call, concluded that primates do not go beneath the surface in their social interactions and do not gain understanding of the goals, perceptions, knowledge and beliefs that guide the actions of others.[181] By 2008, however, having reviewed the recent evidence, they had decided on a "definite yes, chimpanzees do have a theory of mind."[182]

An accumulating number of observations had led them to make this statement. For one thing, when gesturing, chimpanzees are sensitive to where the intended receiver of their communication is looking[183] and will even move in front of the recipient to make sure their communication is seen.[184] Chimpanzees use this skill by concealing their approach to food whose ownership might be disputed. Both chimpanzees and rhesus monkeys have been observed keeping track of what another has seen a moment before – even if this other individual can no longer see it now.[185–188] A more recent experiment took advantage of the preference of chimpanzees for stealing back confiscated food from an opaque container rather than a transparent one – presumably to avoid detection. Researchers arranged both containers to look opaque from the viewpoint of the chimpanzee. However, if previous experience had already informed the chimpanzee that one container was transparent from the viewpoint of the researchers, they tended to avoid it.[189] If the researcher wasn't present, this tendency disappeared. The chimpanzee appeared to be working out what the researchers were thinking.

Although other primates possess some theory of mind, there was one remaining way in which our own species might still differ in kind from other primates. By the age of 3–4 a child can understand that another person has a belief which is false, and be able to predict their behaviour based on this false belief.[186] Until recently, it was thought humans were the only species able to do this. However, using eye-tracking equipment, researchers have studied the gaze of apes watching a human search for a hidden object. When the apes, but not the human, had seen the object be moved to another location, their gaze still anticipated the human searching for it in its original position.[190] The researchers confirmed this behaviour for orangutans and two types of chimpanzee, suggesting other primates can also predict the behaviour of another, even when this is based on a belief that they themselves know is false.

Primates and social learning

Animals can learn from direct experience with the world by exploring the material world or the relationships with others, but many can also learn by watching others doing this. We've already seen how interested primates are in others' business, and how that helps them adapt their strategies according to what others know. This ability to learn from the actions of others – even when these actions are not especially designed to teach or communicate – is called "social learning".[191] It can greatly boost the speed and efficiency by which a whole community can acquire new information or a new skill.[192] It existed well before teaching but it can still play an important role in children's and adults' education (see box below). Social learning means an individual doesn't have to discover everything for themselves – which can be a time-consuming and risky process.

Social learning in education

In education, spoken and written language tend to be the dominant media of learning, but learning through observation still plays an important and under-appreciated role – particularly when language is still developing. For example, toddlers of less than two years old can learn from watching complete strangers who are ignoring them.[193] The power of social learning was also shown amongst an older group of children (aged 3–5 years) who were learning to share. Sharing is an important part of developing friendships, but children are not born with an innate tendency to share and so, one way or another, this important skill must be acquired. A small number of children were extracted from the class and explicitly tutored in how to share the tokens they had won for correct answers during class. Over the next few days, researchers were able to track this behaviour spreading throughout the rest of the group, as the other children imitated the actions of those they observed.[194]

Although younger children are more influenced by peer modelling than older children,[195] observational learning continues to operate in adulthood and is particularly valued in sport.[196]

Non-primate animals are capable of learning from another's response to fear and reward. Animals that learn to fear what they observe others fearing[197] include sheep,[198] rats,[199] cats,[200] monkeys[201] and mice.[202] Fear stimulates a response in others that can easily become associated straightforwardly with, for example, the presence of danger in the neighbourhood. Similarly with reward. A voyeuristic type of reinforcement learning is thought to underpin foraging as a group. In this activity, group members attract the attention of the others when a food patch is discovered – a phenomenon observed amongst birds.[203–207] Primates, however, can also learn from others who display disgust or avoid particular foods, and will change their own food choices accordingly.[208,209] This visceral type of social learning can be seen in human behaviour, when our peers and family influence our own eating habits as young children[210] and as adults.[211]

The day-to-day challenges of primate life also demand a more sophisticated response than just aversion or attraction to something. Primates can watch the actions and experience of another and then replicate it – so demonstrating (and consolidating) their learning about these actions. It is true that a range of non-primate animals, such as octopuses, birds and other mammals, can acquire new skills and social conventions from observing others.[212–214] However, primates have displayed particular competence in this area. Social learning is thought to explain why, for example, very specific behaviours have been reported for some populations of macaques and chimpanzees but not in others. The first and perhaps best-known account was recorded in the 1960s and began with a Japanese macaque called Imo who, when given pieces of sweet potato by the researchers, would wash the sand off the pieces in a nearby stream.[215–217] Around three months after she was first seen doing this, two of Imo's playmates and her mother began to do the same thing. The practice then spread to her playmates' mums and seven other young macaques. The pattern of spread had begun with Imo's closest associates and then their close associates got involved, further suggesting that individuals were learning from each other. Since then, many examples of primates appearing to pick up practices from each other have been recorded.[218] This is clearly significant for the story of our learning brain, since this type of learning appears close to the types of cultural transmission of knowledge achieved by early humans when, for example, producing stone tools. However, when you stop to consider such imitation, it's not immediately obvious how it can happen. When it comes to our own actions, we can learn associations by activating our muscles in different ways and seeing the results. That sort of learning is happening when a baby is kicking its legs and waving its arms. For the actions of another, we don't have the experience of moving their body – so how can we learn the muscle activity required? The mirror neuron system may be part of the answer.

When we observe someone else performing an action, some of our own brain regions activate as if we were performing the action ourselves. This phenomenon has been observed in humans, non-human primates and rodents, and the system enabling it is called the mirror neuron system.

It seems unlikely that animals are born with this system, just the potential to acquire it. In other words, it is a learning tool that is itself learnt. From early on, by experiencing their own movements, animals build associations between seeing their action and the sensing of their bodies during the action – the type of information used to perform it. If they then form associations between their own movements and similar movements

---

Mirror neurons and educational interventions

In Chapter 2 you came across the enactment effect, i.e. the increased learning that is achieved when a learner practices actions relevant to what they are trying to learn. However, increased memory for observing a teacher using actions and gestures has also been measured for both adults and 4–5-year-old children.[219] So, for example, children and adults were more likely to remember the word "stack" had been used if the teacher used this gesture for "stack" when she spoke it:

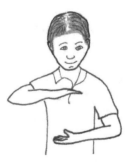

This may best be understood though the notion of mirror neurons – i.e. that regions of the students' brains were activating when observing the teacher as if they were carrying out the actions themselves. This has the potential to enhance memory for the word by expanding its representation in the brain to include networks for sensing and movement.

Understanding more about the underlying neural processes of social learning may be insightful for education. The involvement of the mirror neuron system may help explain why students find moving images beneficial for acquiring skills that involve human movement, such as knot tying, assembly, first-aid procedures, puzzle construction or origami tasks.[220–225] In other types of learning, the transient nature of moving images can often just place greater load on our working memory and make learning more difficult.[226]

carried out by others, then their own performance-related information can be automatically accessed when seeing others' actions. Imitation of a new procedure – like seeing a fellow primate pick a stick and use it as a tool – may just be a matter of activating existing associations for the actions used, in their observed order. Moreover, the information in the brain that gets activated can extend beyond just the sensory, and include ideas such as the purposes for an action. That means the mirror neuron system might also give insight into *why* someone else is doing an action. This is backed up by evidence that shows the mirror neuron system in monkeys and humans appears sensitive to goals, producing different patterns of brain activation when observing others doing the same actions but for different reasons.[227] In short, the mirror neuron system may, to some degree, be an unconscious window into the minds of others. By partly activating our brains as though we are doing the actions ourselves, this system helps us to decode the deeds of those around us and can provide clues as to what's going on in their minds. The existence of the mirror neuron system also helps us understand why certain types of educational interventions are successful (see box on previous page).

Social learning and choosing your role model

One challenge for the social learner is deciding who to learn from. Several factors can decide whether an individual's behaviour gets emulated. These factors include familiarity, how high an individual is in the hierarchy and the number of others who are already copying their behaviour. These factors have been observed influencing social learning in a wide range of animals. For example, social learning is influenced by familiarity amongst fishes and by the pecking order amongst hens.[228,229]

Considering another's expertise when selecting them as a teacher should obviously make your social learning more effective, and humans learn to scrutinise their potential teachers early on. In small-scale human societies, for example, children aged 10 and up prefer to learn from mothers they perceive as more successful or knowledgeable.[230] Non-human primates can also be picky about who they choose to model, which suggests assessment of teachers arrived long before our species evolved. Less knowledgeable chimpanzees, for example, spend more time following successful or informed members of their species than other less knowledgeable chimps.[231,232]

A social bias rather than a social module

Although primates, including ourselves, may appear expert in our social learning, there is probably no social module in the primate brain. Social learning uses the same sorts of processes that the brain requires for other types of learning. All that is required for an animal to specialize in social skills may be a bias towards social inputs from their environment – a tendency to look at eyes and faces, to listen to speech and to exchange signals with others. Even these tendencies, however, can themselves be learnt using the ancient learning systems we encountered in Chapter 3. For example, on the surface, you might think that identifying your best role model is intrinsically different from learning to find the best food source. Both, however, require constantly updating the value of different sources based on prediction error (the difference between the actual and expected outcome). Human studies of brain imaging show similar processes at work in both cases.[233] It seems foraging for food and foraging for information are essentially the same sort of problem, and both problems can be solved using the reinforcement learning system.

Social demands may have driven the growth of the primate brain, but across primate species, performance on social and non-social tasks is highly correlated.[234–237] This points more towards the evolution of a flexible brain – one that has an underlying general intelligence (similar to "general intelligence" or "g" in humans) that can be fairly well predicted by brain size.[234,235] The demand may have been social but the result was an expansion of the primate brain that offered greater general flexibility and intelligence.[168] It may only be the constant application of these abilities in the social domain that creates the impression of a primate brain that is born to be social.

Indeed, primates do surprisingly well on a range of non-social cognitive tests, including the ones we use to assess children's development. For example, many modern primates realise an object continues to exist in its last seen location even when they can no longer see it. At around 18 to 24 months of age, human infants build on a similar type of ability and learn to understand how objects can be hidden inside containers. When the object disappears from a container, they can search where it might have left the container without seeing this happen (so-called "invisible displacement").[238,239] A few other non-human primates have demonstrated they can do this too.[240,241] Some apes are also able to recognise how the amount of a liquid stays the same when it's poured from a long thin glass to a wide short one,[242,243,244] which is a skill that appears to develop quite late in childhood, from around seven years old.[245]

Tools

Amongst examples of primates exploring their physical world, it is their use of tools that stirs the greatest human interest. Perhaps this is because tool-making was, for a long time, considered to be a defining feature of humanness. Also, tools are a very physical and prevalent type of evidence

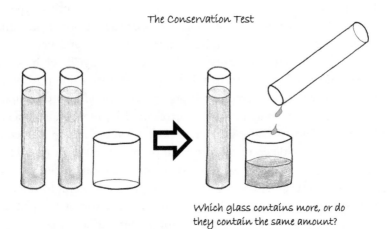

The Conservation Test

Which glass contains more, or do they contain the same amount?

for understanding the human story. We can now assume, however, that the use of tools began well before the arrival of humans. Primates evolved to feed themselves by hand and this, incidentally, has resulted in them being better than other species at handling objects and using their hands to "process" their food.[181] These handling skills, combined with their general interest in the rest of the world, results in apes, capuchins and baboons frequently investigating how their actions impact on new objects they encounter. Through these investigations, they accumulate knowledge suitable for discovering how to use tools more proficiently and to discover new ones.[246,247] Interestingly, in captive situations where non-human primates become exposed to human culture, other monkeys such as macaques also show this ability. Cultural immersion seems a powerful experience for learning, even when the culture belongs to another species. The big tool-users, however, are the chimpanzees. They use tools regularly in the wild, employing leaves to clean and protect food, and sticks and stones to intimidate and injure others, as well as to reach and extract nourishment.

This use of tools, and interest in the processes involved, may help some primates acquire and apply the idea of cause and effect when using objects to reach food. Chimpanzees can, for example, work out the location of food on a balance beam according to its "weight", choosing whichever end moves lower, despite having no previous experience of a balance beam.[248] Apes and capuchin monkeys can even infer which cup contains a piece of food based on whether they hear a sound when the cups are shaken. So, when a primate picks up a stick to extract food, their strategy is probably not just a trial-and-error approach of "what fits in this hole?", but may include knowledge of how an object can cause an effect in terms of its properties ("it needs to have this size, shape, solidity, connectedness and rigidity"). Primate tool-use has also contradicted a popular notion that all non-human animals are "stuck in time",[249] with no ability to plan. Orangutans and bonobos can learn to save a tool by taking it with them, in anticipation of its use up to 14 hours later.[250,251] Tool-use, however, varies greatly across primate species and, amongst non-human primates who use tools, it can often be very sporadic. Mostly, it seems to appear spontaneously and then disappear, with no sense that skills are ever accumulated and dispersed. Assuming tool-use is spread by social learning, this suggests a significant gap between the social learning abilities of human and non-human primates.

Hitting the limits

Even with shrewd decisions about who to learn from, there are clear limits to what non-human primates can achieve through their social learning. If you are a non-human primate, you won't find it easy to learn from the actions of another. For one thing, your teacher will appear very uninterested in your learning. They will not deliberately repeat any stages in the action that you have missed. They may even, in an oblivious fashion, turn their back on you and obscure your view entirely. On top of that, you will need to be present just when and where the required information is being acted out. These barriers to learning would be overcome by a new type of primate arriving in Chapter 5.

Note

i Carpolestid plesiadapiform (*Carpolestes simpsoni*).

5

HOMO – THE COOPERATIVE SOCIAL LEARNER

A 6000 KM SCAR runs down our planet's surface. It starts in Lebanon's Beqaa Valley, and travels through Ethiopia, dividing to travel around Lake Victoria on both sides before re-joining in Tanzania. Finally, it forks into Zimbabwe and Mozambique in South Africa.

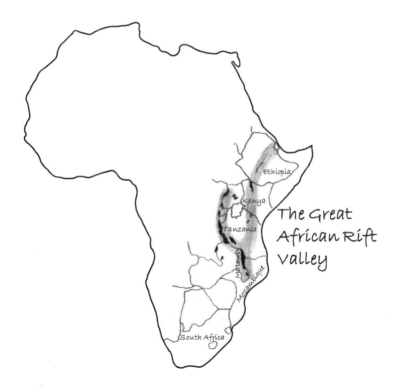

The Great African Rift Valley

As the scar travels south, smaller cracks branch off into other countries and, all along, its route is signposted by lakes. Geologists believe this dramatic wound was started by a "super plume" of molten rock that arose 30 Myr from deep underneath South Africa, close to the core of the Earth. When this super plume burst forth, floods of molten basalt poured out to create the plateaus on either side of the valley. Continental drift then tugged these plateaus in opposite directions. This resulted in a further thinning of the Earth's crust in this region, and more volcanic activity followed as the continents of Asia and Africa tore themselves apart. A series of seismic and fiery episodes were punctuated by periods of relative peace. Apart from the immediate effects of earthquakes, ash and lava from all the volcanic explosions and activity, the long-term effect was an uplift of regions around the rift.[252] Winds, atmospheric moisture and rainfall changed, resulting in a less tropical and much drier climate[253] and periods (between 8 and 2 Myr) when grasslands were spreading and woodlands were receding.[254,255]

These episodes of geological violence dealt death and devastation when they occurred, but they may also have created a crucible for evolution. Environmental change had prompted evolutionary adaptation in the past but, here in the Rift Valley, change was now occurring at a much faster rate. This was the setting for a critical chapter in human evolution, and it's here that we find evidence of the earliest hominins: the *Homo* genus that would eventually diversify into our own species.

Hominins

Hominins are great apes with distinctive features for surviving a drier climate of grassland and savannah, rather than woodland. They have an erect posture, an ability to move on two feet (bipedalism) and larger brains. There were once many different types of hominins but we represent the only surviving species. Genetic estimates of when humans and chimpanzees split from their common ancestor provide a rough indication of when the hominin line began – around 6.3 to 8 Myr.[256,257] This wide range reflects uncertainty in genetic estimates but also the possibility that the genetic changes may have been spread over millions of years.[256]

The earliest fossil evidence of these changes remains frustratingly partial. The oldest contender[i] for the hominin title dates from 7 Myr and was found in Chad.[258,259] However, this consists of just a distorted cranium and two jaw bones, making its identification very difficult.[260] Another specimen,[ii] found in Northern Kenya, includes a set of molar teeth and part of a thigh bone.[261] These are potentially interesting, because modern humans have thick tooth enamel and their habit of walking on two feet comes with a thickening of the thigh bone at the top and bottom of its neck. Although the specimen had the thick tooth enamel, we now know this is not exclusive to humans and scans of the thigh have not been able to confirm the thickening of its neck.[260] A more complete hominin candidate[iii] was found in Ethiopia and has been dated to around 4.4 Myr. This creature appeared capable of walking both on all fours and occasionally on two feet, and was uniquely adapted for moving through trees and across the ground. In this small-brained specimen, the canine (biting) teeth are reduced and similar in size for males and females, suggesting less conflict between males, more pair bonding and more parental care. In other words, considerable changes in social behaviour were occurring well before the arrival of big brains. However, it must be said that most of what this adds up to is a huge question mark about hominin evolution in the period 7–4 Myr.[155]

Things become clearer after **4 Myr**, when we find the earliest undisputed hominin fossils. These belong to the *Australopithecus* group. From 3.85 Myr, we have over 300 specimens of *Australopithecus afarensis* in East Africa, including the well-known "Lucy" specimen from Ethiopia. This primate still had an ape-like face with a flat nose and lower projecting jaw, long arms and curved fingers for tree climbing, and its brain was still only one-third the size of a modern human. But it also possessed small canine teeth and regularly walked upright on two legs like we do. This species represents a plateau in evolution that survived unchanged for more than 900,000 years – about four times longer than presently achieved by our own species. Although still small-brained, *A. afarensis* possessed bones strongly adapted for long-distance walking, allowing access to a wider range of food resources.

Hello *Homo*!

Somewhere between 1.9 and 2.5 Myr, *Australopithecus* diverged to produce the first members of the *Homo* genus. This range, however, again reflects uncertainty and another break in the fossil record. There is a frustratingly small number of fossil specimens from this period to tell us when and how the critical changes came about[262] and the story may, anyway, have been a "long and fuzzy" transition.[263] In contrast, there is a richness of fossils dated to between 1.8 and 1.9 Myr. These show that diversity in East Africa amongst hominins was peaking. We find fossils in Tanzania, Kenya, Ethiopia, Malawi and South Africa showing at least three *Homo* species[iv] in existence at the same time.[264] *H. habilis* had an estimated brain size of around 50% larger than *Australopithecus*, and *H. erectus* had a 20% larger brain again and 15% larger body than the other types of *Homo* alive at the time.

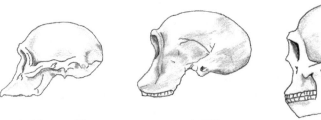
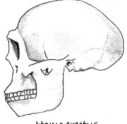

Australopithecus africanus   Homo habilis   Homo erectus

Bigger brains and bodies point to changes in lifestyle, and there are other new features that suggest primate evolution was now emphasising a more flexible approach. The shoulder could perform throwing,[265] the lower body allowed long-distance running[266] and hominin teeth could now eat meat as well as vegetation.[267] All these features point to a wider set of strategies for sourcing food. The new bipedal primates displayed a range of eating habits and were dispersing outwards from their origins, so encountering new habitats and new potential food sources.[268] A more flexible approach to life meant greater social cooperation with more choices and more decisions to make. In short, life was becoming more complicated, favouring the acquisition and application of more cognitive skills, and further increase in costly brain tissue. This trend towards flexibility may not sound radical, but it's an odd twist in the evolutionary tale. Generally, evolution tends towards more efficient design through "speciation for specialisation". So why was this a good time and place to be a generalist rather than a specialist?

Flexibility valley

It seems likely that it was the geological upheavals in the Rift Valley that drove the evolution and dispersal of bigger-brained non-specialist primates. This move towards expensive generalisation was even more remarkable by occurring multiple times and, broadly speaking, in the same geological region of our planet. As well as *H. erectus* and several of its ancestors, the East African Rift System has also provided remains of the first anatomically modern humans.[269]

Rather than a coincidence, the more reasonable explanation for all this genetic innovation is down to the very special nature of this region in prehistory. Shifting tectonic plates helped create the Rift Valley alongside mountains and basins suitable for lakes, but also produced heaps of volcanic activity. This would have had a big effect on the region's weather and water cycle. The unique geology of the Rift Valley, combined with the Earth's orbit around the Sun, is thought to have produced extreme climate variability with cycles lasting 400,000 or 800,000 years. Each of these periods comprised 4–5 wet–dry cycles in which lakes would grow rapidly for a few hundred years, fill most of the Rift Valley for a few thousand years and then rapidly and erratically disappear.[270] Following this, another long dry period of thousands of years would come about. These wet–dry cycles occurred until around 800 Kyr when other influences, such as global glaciation, began to take over.[271]

This inconsistent environment provided a novel genetic testing ground in which different hominin species were pursuing different approaches to survival, including generalising vs. specialising. Some descendants of *Australopithecus* specialised in eating tougher vegetation during the lean times, while others (*Homo*) tended towards a package of changes that provided flexibility. Bipedalism allowed for long-distance movement to new food sources, but an increasing tendency towards eating meat also supported increasingly larger brains. These bipedal hominins were able to move greater distances, and became more varied in their diet, tooluse and social cooperation, so achieving access to a broader range of food resources.[263,272,273] In other words, rather than evolving to fit one change, they evolved greater ability to respond to change itself.

Flexibility, of course, did not arrive all at once. Rather, following our principle of gradualism, it evolved slowly over time. It was a natural emerging process and, indeed, some of the flexibility features we associate with being "human" were already emerging in *Australopithecus*. Some fossils of larger specimens of this species show similar hind-leg proportions and as much bipedal advantage as smaller specimens of *Homo*, and there is even evidence of tool-use as well. New analytical techniques and recent finds suggest that the one consistent difference, present from the earliest fossil records of *Homo*, was one of the overall size of the body and brain. All the different species of *Homo* are, on average, larger than *Australopithecus*, indicating a more nutrition-rich diet and predicting the potential to travel over a greater range to access more diverse habitats and food resources. The need for flexibility, linked to variability in climate, is thought to have driven these general increases in *Homo* body and brain size.

What sort of flexibility was key?

Although a bigger body extends travel opportunities, the advantage of a bigger brain is more questionable. Given the expense of neural tissue in terms of energy, some serious justification is needed. What sort of information processing was *Homo* doing that could have been so important? In terms of material evidence, we can see an increase in the use of tools, but tool-use alone appears a poor explanation. This is, after all, something that smaller-brained primates (and many non-primates) can do. It may, however, provide a clue. Tools were mostly being used for gaining valuable resources through ventures such as hunting that benefit from a coordinated group effort.[274–277] The distance that raw material was being carried to construct the tools was also on the increase, from 1 km by 2 Myr, to as far as 13 km by 1.6 Myr.[278] It is the social flexibility that lies behind the new lifestyle, such as the cooperation and social coordination required to resource, construct and use tools, that most likely drove brain expansion. Social competencies are needed to achieve these things, including a sense of group and being able to negotiate the roles within it. This means getting beyond the level of spontaneous one-to-one interactions. Patterns of social trust were required based on a communal sense of what's to be expected.

The genus *Homo* was carving out a niche based on overcoming ecological challenges with teamwork. This teamwork required a flexible processing of social information – a constant monitoring and reworking of alliances and social information – such that social learning would have become a key factor influencing the fitness of the group and so driving cerebral expansion. This expansion, though driven by social factors, would have provided an increase in general intelligence – so adding to success when tackling physical as well as social problems. General intelligence remains an important factor impacting on our success today (see box opposite).

Over geological time, we can make some assumptions about *Homo*'s increase in flexible intelligence based on the increased size of fossilised brain cavities and, therefore, the size of the brain. It would be wrong, however, to assume the intelligence of an individual is all about biological inheritance. There is a range of findings that confirm intelligence can be increased by environmental influences in our modern world. Researchers have reported improvements for short interventions ranging from "brain training" to playing off-the-shelf video games, music lessons and a programme of problem-solving and creativity. It also seems that these effects are not restricted to children, so reflecting the lifelong plasticity of the brain (see also Chapter 10). If relatively brief interventions have an influence, it is not surprising that a host of longer-term issues, many linked to socio-economic background, also have impact. Positive factors for children's intelligence include permanent housing, degree of parental education, good-quality experience in pre-school care and high-quality relationships within the home, with negative factors including parental neglect.[279]

General intelligence

General intelligence is something that has been measured in many species, but its prehistorical significance for *Homo* may be reflected in its continuing high regard today. It has been argued that general intelligence should be divided into two flavours: *crystallised intelligence* based on directly applying knowledge from previous situations, and *flexible intelligence*, which is our ability to cope with new situations we have not experienced before.[280] Flexible intelligence is commonly considered a strong predictor of success in today's world, both academically and professionally.[281,282]

In a typical test of flexible intelligence, participants are asked to identify the pattern (from eight alternatives) that continues a sequence. The answer to this example is at the bottom of this box:

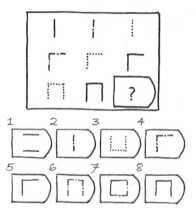

The answer to the example above is number 6.

These environmental effects on intelligence also imply the possibility of a genetic–environmental loop that can make genetic changes more impactful. Genetic influences on intelligence do not show themselves strongly from the outset, although by around eight years of age they explain half of the modern variability we see today, and this rises to around three-quarters during adulthood.[283] This late genetic influence may be due to genetic differences becoming amplified by how they influence an individual to create the environment around them, which then further influences development of their intelligence. It is arguable, therefore, how much the outcome of an intelligence test should be categorised as genetic – in the sense that it's fixed by our biology. The genetic–environmental feedback loop would also have boosted the rewards of cerebral expansion in prehistory, especially if these were being applied in communal projects. As our ancestors developed greater intelligence, this would be reflected in the challenges they shared together, providing the type of stimulus that could develop their mental abilities further, and generating a flexible intelligence "bonus".

That all sounds great – but greater flexibility did not guarantee a competitive edge. Ultimately, the survival of a generalist approach would rest on a simple question: can the increased food provided by a flexible, bigger brain justify the additional energy that this new brain demands? When conditions were changeable enough, the answer appears to be "yes". A study of temperature change over the last 2 million years showed that its variability predicts changes in *Homo* brain size.[284] (The same study speculated that, if temperature variation drove the evolution of bigger brains, fossil skulls found further from the equator would indicate larger brains – due to greater seasonal changes. Results confirmed that this was the case.) The finer details in the pattern of brain enlargement reflect the appearances of each new species in Africa while, in Eurasia, step changes in brain size at 100 Kyr and at 200–400 Kyr appear linked to migrations of these new African hominin species into Eurasia.[285]

Extended family life – a new impetus for collaboration and cooperation

If flexible teamwork was a driving force in human evolution, then there is a puzzle that needs solving. Our closest genetic relative is the chimpanzee, but chimps don't display the sorts of tendencies that could give way to *Homo*-style collaboration. Like all primates, chimpanzees are social creatures but they use their social skills in a self-serving manner.[286,287] Apart from our own species, great apes tend to leave each other to look for their own food (even the infants) and, although they will occasionally allow others to take it, they rarely share voluntarily.[288] Great ape mothers generally receive no help in rearing their young and usually only offer scraps to their offspring.[289] At first sight, this behaviour suggests our shared ancestors may not have possessed the "cognitive platform" needed for launching *Homo*-like teamwork.

The answer to the riddle may be childcare. At some point, the *Homo* line adopted cooperative breeding – a tendency we don't share with chimpanzees or other great apes generally. Although there are massive cultural differences in human approaches to child rearing, there are no human cultures that generally expect a mother to raise their child unaided.[290–292] More evidence for cooperative breeding comes from present-day hunter-gatherers who, arguably, still encounter some of the everyday challenges and conditions faced by early *Homo*. These groups survive through intense cooperation and interdependence, including the sharing of meat.[293,294] When hunting is unproductive, returns are supplemented by gathering foods, and there is communal building of shelters using socially learnt skills.[295] Mothers do not raise their infants independently but receive systematic and flexible direct help through babysitting, carrying and feeding, as well as indirect help through material resources. "Stand-in" mums who are often grandmothers and older siblings (technically referred to as "allomothers") increase the growth and survival chances of the children.[292,296]

Over a million years ago, shared childcare may have encouraged the traits and behaviours required to launch a whole new level of social learning and, ultimately, something similar to human collaborative culture. Chimpanzees may not be cooperative breeders, but there are other primates who have convergently evolved with *Homo* to provide this parenting approach.[297] These are the marmosets and tamarins, which all tend to live in family groups around a breeding pair, with adult helpers and infants. Helpers are usually adult offspring of the breeding pair who are not reproducing,[298] but helpers may also include unrelated individuals.[299–301] Dads and helpers contribute to rearing the infants by carrying them and later sharing their food with them. During the first 5–6 weeks, infants of these species must be carried all the time. Although mothers are the primary carers at night, infants can often spend most of the day with the allomothers, returning to the mother only for breastfeeding.[302,303] To keep them safe, infants are never put down until the next caregiver picks them up, and are always handed over directly. In some respects, food sharing can sometimes appear like other non-human primates with infants begging and adults tolerating, but the frequency of this food sharing is much higher, and adults end up sharing most of their food with the younger generation.[304,305] Also, unlike other non-human primates, there are frequent examples of adults proactively offering food, who hold it in their outstretched hand, make a specific sound and then wait for it to be taken.[288,306,307]

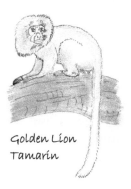

Golden Lion
Tamarin

Since cooperative breeding can be achieved with much smaller brains than ours, it cannot, on its own, explain brain expansion. Cooperative breeding may, however, have got the ball rolling by providing a mental "platform" for *Homo*-style teamwork. Just being tolerant of others is critical in cooperative breeding, because otherwise tensions can disrupt the transferring of infants between caregivers – with potentially lethal consequences for the infant. Paying positive attention and monitoring the location and behaviour of others is important too.[308] One individual needs to know when another is getting tired of carrying an infant and needs to be relieved, and monitoring helps when negotiating the movements and timing needed for safely transferring the infant. Finally, there's good evidence of tamarins and marmosets actively setting out to help others. All these qualities vary across different primate species according to the extent of their cooperative breeding.[297,309]

The oxytocin switch

It may seem incredible that we must look to such a distant part of our primate ancestry to find behaviours we now understand as critical for human evolution. How can the marmosets and tamarins share their cooperative parenting habits with us, and the additional skills associated with them, while our closest genetic relative (the chimpanzee) shows so little of these tendencies? However, a relatively simple genetic change may be responsible.[310,311]

Oxytocin is both a neurotransmitter and a hormone that is involved with the processes of social bonding in mammals. It has an ancient role in reproduction and mother–infant interaction (in birth, producing milk and parenting) but it can become involved in other types of social interaction too.[312,313] A simple change in this oxytocin production enables more positive interaction between all in-group members – of the type required for cooperative breeding. For example, humans who sniff a dose of oxytocin show greater trust[314,315] and generosity[316] towards others in their group. In marmosets, increasing oxytocin encourages fathers to share their food more.[317] In family living, the natural oxytocin levels of adult marmosets are synchronised, and vary in a way that correlates with their positive social behaviour within the group.[313] Most striking is the effect of increasing this hormone in rhesus macaques. These primates are not cooperative breeders and are much more individualistic and tyrannical in their behaviour. Although normally unable to share their food even with their own infants, after receiving additional oxytocin these primates can give to each other, even without receiving any personal reward in return.[318] All this suggests that the basis of active social cooperation lies dormant in the primate brain, except amongst those species whose oxytocin levels allow its expression. Oxytocin effectively switches on the bias that causes us to positively attend to those within our group.[319] (It is worth noting, however, that oxytocin is not all about love and peace. It can increase dishonesty that serves the whole group[320] and generate less positive effects towards out-groups.)[321–323]

A simple increase in oxytocin levels can help create a more intimate social environment in which more positive attention gets paid to each other's behaviour and needs, and this can support a more cooperative style of social learning. The sociality that accompanies an increase in oxytocin levels includes, for example, less aversion to angry faces. It seems reasonable that this would help such expressions to be interpreted more deeply rather than just be avoided. These and other effects, such as reducing social stress, suggest oxytocin can increase the opportunities for individuals to learn from each other.

The oxytocin switch may help explain why tamarins and marmosets achieve higher scores in a range of social skills compared with other primates whose brains are 4–6 times larger but who do not cooperatively breed. These skills include social (observational) learning, vocal communication, gaze-following, perspective-taking and cooperative problem-solving.[324] Greater collaboration is also shown in duties not involving infants such as the defence of territory and resources,[325–327] and also the harvesting of large fruits and vegetables.[328] For example, tamarins work jointly to open a pod of Inga (a white-flowered shrub that produces large (~30 cm) "bean-like" pods of seeds) and then take turns waiting and feeding on the seeds before jointly opening another.[328]

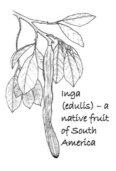

Inga
(edulis) – a
native fruit
of South
America

The birth of teaching

The social skills for cooperative breeding, and the environment they create, don't just aid the receiving of information. They can also help an individual alter their behaviour to help transfer information, i.e. to become more like a teacher. Many primates give food calls when finding a food patch or large food item and these calls can help infants feed. Tamarins emit staccato chirps when they find food, but also encourage the young to approach and take food offered from their hands. In a study of wild golden lion tamarins, only the young approached when adults offered prey and made these calls, something adults were more likely to do when the prey was difficult to handle.[329] As these young tamarins got older and more skilled at finding and handling food themselves, the calls decreased and their context changed. The adult, when finding prey nearby, would now resist capturing the prey themselves and instead just call and wait. This allowed the developing tamarins to arrive and try their hand, foraging themselves for the prey and devouring it as soon as they found it.[330] A laboratory study under more controlled conditions has reported similar behaviour amongst cotton-top tamarins.[331]

Educators reading this book may spot several teacher-like aspects to the above description of tamarin behaviour. The tamarin teacher is differentiating its approach according to the ability of the learner, selecting a rich learning context and a "teachable moment". A good teacher also monitors learning and, in both these studies, the adults are progressively providing less assistance, as if responding to the improving abilities of their young students. This ability to attend to someone else's receipt of information might be considered as a foundational mental skill for building culture. When we attend to the significance of our behaviour for another, we become culturally empowered to shape the thoughts of those around us.

Towards a basis for cultural learning

Of course, we have no proof that tamarins are deliberately attempting to shape the minds of their infants, and some have argued that their social abilities are not unique to cooperative breeders or necessarily demanding.[332] However, such arguments, even if upheld, don't seem to undermine how significant cooperative breeding may have been for our evolution: it still had the potential to tip the balance of probabilities towards making learning more likely. This makes it possible that a modest evolutionary change, such as a sustained increase in oxytocin levels, could have helped lay the foundation for a cultural, rather than purely social, *Homo* niche. In its most primitive sense, the word "cultural" here need not refer to material or even spoken culture, but simply to behaviours that take account of another's attention. This "attention to others' attention" is a common aspect of all human culture. Powerful cultural artefacts – whether a piece of jewelery or a religious symbol – appear to have one thing in common: they are created in a way that is mindful of others' attention and they can usually capture it very effectively. This helps to make them useful tools for communication and learning.

In a potential learner–teacher interaction, "attention to others' attention" can lead to greater likelihood of social learning in different ways but these all generally involve the *active influence* of a role model. In a further study of tamarins, for example, learning achieved between adults was predicted by the degree of attention to the teacher but also the frequency with which the teacher demonstrated the skill.[333] This approximates to the familiar concept of teaching for those who practise and research education. It echoes a model of learning that was first formulated by Vygotsky (see box overleaf), who argued that the mental abilities of children are shaped by interactions with others in their culture, or with artefacts and symbols created by others. We are familiar with these ideas in terms of child development, but they also now appear a central part of how our species evolved, a view supported by studies of other non-human species.[334]

The cultural intelligence hypothesis

An inclination towards following the attention of others can result in learning about the rewards that interest them, which may also interest you. This makes further following more likely, allowing the opportunities to interpret and learn more. In this way, a non-genetic "ratchet effect" would have begun. It is hard to find clear evidence of this "learning to learn" ability in tamarins or marmosets, which may reflect the constraints of their small brain, but we do see this effect in humans (see box on p. 98).

Recently, the idea of a cultural ratchet effect has extended the social brain hypothesis to become the "cultural intelligence hypothesis".[168] This considers social learning, rather than just social behaviour, as the key feature of the niche that the evolving *Homo* genus was beginning to occupy. It was social learning that placed greater demands on mental abilities such as general intelligence. Social learning may sound too "specific" to impact on general mental ability, but it chiefly depends on those underlying learning processes that are not social. Across species of birds and primates[235,335] and across individuals within a species,[336,337] abilities to learn in social and

How attention to others' attention can support learning and teaching

Teachers attend to and capture the attention of potential learners

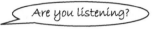

Are you listening?

The ideas of Vygotsky underlie much educational thinking, including his concept of the Zone of Proximal Development (ZPD) – the gap between what is to be known and what is known already. Vygotsky believed that a teacher should identify what a student presently understands and, through social interaction in the ZPD, support the learner to construct new understanding – a process now referred to as "scaffolding".

In its simplest form, such scaffolding might begin with attention to the learner's attention. In the teaching of a skill, *monitoring* where the student is

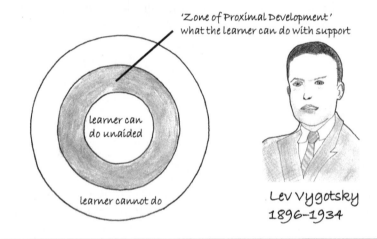

'Zone of Proximal Development'
what the learner can do with support

learner can do unaided

learner cannot do

Lev Vygotsky
1896–1934

non-social contexts are correlated. Doing well in one type will probably mean doing well in the other type. Even the common octopus and red-footed tortoise, which are solitary animals and far removed from us, are capable of social learning,[338] which also points to its rather general nature. What made *Homo* good at social learning may simply have been an enlarged general processing capacity and an inclination to cooperatively breed.

Both our genetic biases towards certain inputs, and the learning processes these biases encourage, are "grist to the mills" of cultural transmission.[191] But in the complex human world, these operate through the culture they attending can provide clues about where the student is going right or wrong – or what they have learnt and still must learn (i.e. their ZPD). A teacher who wishes to make a student conscious of new information must also be aware of when they have *captured* the student's attention before attempting to introduce new information. Rehearsal of this process of monitoring and capturing the learner's attention can improve the abilities of both teacher and learner to achieve the *shared* attention required for most teacher–student interactions.

Learners benefit from attending to and capturing the attention of potential teachers

Please Miss!

Attending to and capturing the attention of those around you is also an important skill for a budding learner. For example, cooperative play allows young children to acquire and rehearse a range of important social skills. Gaining the attention of potential playmates has a direct bearing on how many of these play opportunities come along. In one experiment, researchers provided children (7–9 years old) with plastic figures and three landscapes to play with them in (a castle, tower and forest).[339] Some of the characters possessed audio (e.g. the dragon roared). As expected, children frequently make attention bids to one another during the session (e.g. showing the toy or seeking eye contact). However, they were more likely to capture the attention of the other child when possessing a toy that emitted audio, and these bids resulted in more cooperative play. Here, the increased capacity to capture another's attention was achieved artificially, but it illustrates the potential importance of a child's own skills in capturing shared attention as a first step in cooperative play. It is also an example of how material culture can play a role in this process – something we'll return to in Chapter 6.

help create, and so are likely to be influenced by this culture. It has been shown, for example, that Western Caucasians divide their attention more equally between the eyes and mouth than East Asians, who focus more on the eyes.[340] This has influence on how easily different emotions are recognised, reflecting how input biases become tuned by cultural environments. More tuning to a certain stimulus is likely to result in more of that stimulus arriving. This is one way in which social learning quickly becomes characterised by the culture that supports it, both in terms of its processes and the content of the learning.

The rewards of shared attention – and learning to learn

Researchers have shown that infants will occasionally notice a parent looking towards what he/she is holding, and will then tend to look in that direction.[341] It's known that in children, as well as adults, spontaneous shared attention activates those brain regions that process reward and are bound up with our motivation.[342] This supports the idea that learning to follow someone's eye-gaze – a key social skill that can lead to shared attention – can be achieved through the type of reinforcement learning involving the basal ganglia[343] that we came across in Chapter 3. When we have learnt to gaze-follow, then we can much more efficiently learn from a teacher – so this is an important step in learning to learn. However, while all primates (and vertebrates) possess basal ganglia, the opportunities for learning to follow eye-gaze should arise more frequently in cooperatively breeding communities, where resources are shared.

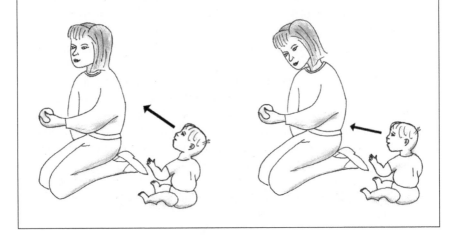

Tool school

Tool-use may have improved incidentally as a result of *Homo*'s socially-driven brain expansion but, as a potentially cooperative activity, it may also have favoured a more cooperative approach to learning. Whether we should think of it as more cause or more effect, the improving quality of tool-making tells us social learning was on the rise. The earliest signs of a stone tool industry (with tools sharing the same form and function) is amongst *Australopithecus* and early *Homo*. This early type of tool is called "Oldowan", which is a term derived from the Olduvai Gorge in Tanzania, a Rift Valley site where the first tools of this type were found. Oldowan tools were made by a process of "knapping". This involves striking a round hammer stone on a core rock to produce a curved fracture with sharp edges that can be used for many different purposes. The chip that comes away is called the flake. The core rock can be anything that maintains a sharp edge, such as obsidian, basalt or flint. To reduce the core, there are specific strategies and rules governing how and where the next removal of stone should occur relative to the previous ones.[344] By 2.5 Myr, knappers were removing 70 or more flakes from the core and demonstrating a systematic approach: the ability to plan, to maintain striking angles, to repair and to recycle.[345,346]

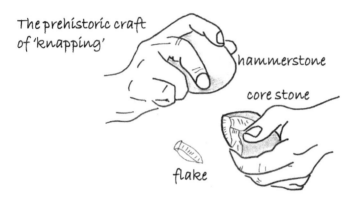

The prehistoric craft of 'knapping'

hammerstone

core stone

flake

Fully-formed Oldowan tools may have arisen in the Rift Valley around 2.6 Myr, with dispersion outwards such that by 2.0–1.7 Myr they were present throughout much of East Africa,[347–349] North Africa[350] and South Africa.[351] Comparison of tools found at different sites suggests their makers possessed a similar set of mental abilities. More interestingly, the same use of specific strategies seems to be getting used in almost all places close enough for some cultural connection. It seems unlikely these practices were always being invented over again, and much more likely they spread via a process of learning. That said, the learning was not very accumulative.[352] There may have been variations in approach but nothing that added up to technological progress beyond a least-effort production of sharp edges. Once dispersed, the tool-making of early *Homo* entered a state of stasis.

At around 1.7 Myr, a fresh wave of innovation arrived. The new Acheulean tools boasted hand-axes in which the stone was worked symmetrically and on both sides.[353] The makers of these tools followed several stages and were including materials other than stone. These more sophisticated skills were also being passed down the generations. Similar tools are found close to the sources of the stone, suggesting social groups were communicating their strategies more efficiently to each other.

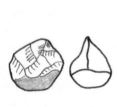
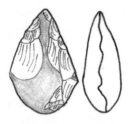
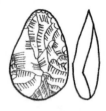

 Oldowan   Early Acheulean   Late Acheulean

This upgrade in technology hints at an upgrade in teaching and learning capability – and the emergence of early spoken language. A different type of tool was arriving that was to prove much more powerful than any piece of stone.

Notes

i *Sahelanthropus tchadensis.*
ii *Orrorin tugenensis.*
iii *Ardipithecus ramidus.*
iv *H. habilis, H. rudolfensis* and *H. erectus.*

6

SPEECH

HE FOUNDATIONS OF CULTURE were already being practised by **1.8 Myr**, a little while after the *Homo* genus had diverged into species that included *H. habilis* and *H. erectus*. At this point, it appears that hominins were cooperatively breeding, hunting large game and protecting their kills. They were successfully gathering the valuable but hard-to-use underground parts of plants and using stone tools to get at meat. All these activities required a collaborative flexible approach, arising from an interest in each other's behaviour and attention. These foundations would provide the all-important platform for launching language.

But language did not arrive suddenly[354] and this is reflected in the rate at which technology was advancing or, rather, not advancing. In some respects, *H. habilis* (or "handy man") achieved a great step forward in terms of technology, using its 600-cc brain to acquire the least-energy approach to tool-making called Oldowan. As well as being effective, it was simple enough to be passed between users across great distances and down genera-tions using whatever communication skills were available. However, the fact that Oldowan progress essentially "froze" for 700,000 years tells us these communication skills were probably limited (see box overleaf). Any simple developments in tool-making were getting lost as quickly as they came along. A telling increase in innovation can be seen in the so-called "Acheulean" tools of *H. erectus*, whose remains (from around 1.9 Myr) indicate a brain size of about 800–1000 cc. This upgrade in tool-making suggests *H. erectus* may have developed the beginnings of a language or

The importance of symbolic language for learning – even in our early prehistory

The extent to which new skills were being transferred in prehistory tells us something about how they were being learnt, because different ways of learning vary in their efficiency. A recent experiment demonstrated this. The research involved chains of up to 10 adults trying to pass on Oldowan stone knapping skills from one to the other.[355] The goal was to produce good-quality flakes, which requires careful attention to edges and angles. Each chain used one of five different approaches to transmit the necessary information: 1. Reverse engineering (just studying the outcomes produced by another), 2. Imitation/emulation (observing the skill performed by another), 3. Basic teaching (demonstrating in a way that was attentive to the learner's attention – ensuring they had a clear view and slowing their actions to help the learner), 4. Gestural teaching (using gestures but without verbal sound) and 5. Verbal teaching (teachers and learners were also allowed to speak).

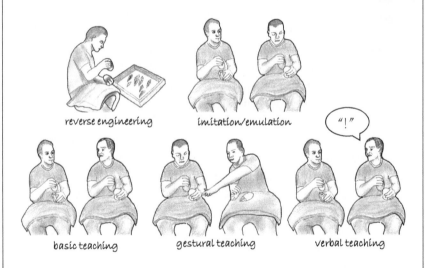

reverse engineering   imitation/emulation

basic teaching   gestural teaching   verbal teaching

The results showed that total flake quality only improved with gestural or verbal teaching. It seems even a purely practical and concrete task can benefit when a teacher uses symbols. Some early language development would – whether based on gesture or speech – have boosted teaching power, making it more likely that some new habits that were culturally favoured could be retained by communities. The findings illustrate how the 700,000-year stasis of Oldowan technology may reflect a lack of symbol use by *H. habilis*, while the quality and progression of Acheulean technology suggests some form of gestural or verbal proto-language was emerging amongst *H. erectus*.

"proto-language". The brain of *H. erectus* is still small compared with our own, indicating less general intelligence and simpler social organisation but, aided by whatever proto-language it possessed, this species dispersed itself across the old world. This would have been no mean feat. Occasionally, cold glacial events allowed the usual monsoon and tropical rain systems to weaken, making the more northerly deserts more passable. However, crossing the desert barrier of northern Africa and the southern Middle East would still have been an immense challenge for this species.[356] The existence of early speech would help explain how, by 1.7 Myr, the *H. erectus* species had spread out of Africa across Eurasia to China.[357]

The arrival of *H. sapiens* – and (close) friends

The creative forces of the Rift Valley continued to impact on human evolution, with further increases in *Homo* brain expansion. Amongst its many treasures, the Rift provides some of the oldest evidence of *H. heidelbergensis*.[358–360] This species had a skull size range that overlaps with modern humans, and is thought to be the last common ancestor of both *Homo neanderthalis* and *Homo sapiens*.[361]

The earliest collection of features that might identify our own species (*H. sapiens*) has been found in Ethiopia.[362–364] The fossil record suggests *H. sapiens* gradually accumulated its modern features from between **200 Kyr** to our Great Expansion out of Africa around 45–60 Kyr.[365] This Great Expansion brought the *H. sapiens* lineage back into contact with those other species who had already left, which included the Neanderthals and another group of ancestors called the Denisovans.[366] The increasing spread of *H. sapiens* and the extinction of these other types of primate has sometimes been portrayed as a type of battle that powered evolutionary progress, but it is important to resist this idea. Generally, evolutionary science doesn't "do" the popular idea of progress. Indeed, based on comparisons of modern DNA with those of ancient Neanderthals[367] and Denisovans,[368] there is an unexpected twist to the whole story. It now appears we interbred with these other primates and still possess part of their genetic matter. This pours cold water on the idea of a heated battle between species. Instead, according to our biological definition of "species" in Chapter 1, Neanderthals, Denisovans and ourselves are all variants of the one same species. This species must have originally arrived from Africa around 300–700 Kyr, prior to diverging into its variants.[367,369–374]

One ancient language?

Analysis of modern speech suggests there was once a single, common ancestral language.[375] Since all modern human populations maintain complex spoken language abilities, this language may have been well developed amongst *H. sapiens* before or during our Great Expansion.[365] However, tracking the spread of our species through language families is much more difficult than using genetic groupings. For one thing, language changes very rapidly, so that two populations which previously shared the same language can become incomprehensible to each other within 1000 years. One analysis of language, in line with the genetic analysis, has identified an African origin for *H. sapiens* followed by a dispersion outwards[376] – but debate continues as to whether we can really hear this "Out-of-Africa" echo in the words we speak today.[377]

More concretely, at 45 Kyr, we do see sudden bursts of cultural complexity. There are more sophisticated tools, paintings, sculptures and engravings that reflect a more modern use of spoken communication. The creation of spoken language, from a time without abstract symbols, had taken at least around 2 million years. In fact, given the gap in the fossil record before this time, it probably took even longer than this. With the aid of new insights into the modern human mind and brain, we can begin to identify the stages by which language might have gradually developed, even if the timing of these stages is more uncertain.

Which language came first – gesture or speech?

Although the arrival of modern spoken language has been so significant for learning and for history, the evolutionary idea of "gradualism" suggests we are looking for undramatic origins. We need to find a beginning that we might scarcely recognise as language at all. We are looking for processes that would allow language to emerge seamlessly from a more ordinary "platform" of mental ability.

In addition to our social tendencies and general intelligence, another important part of this platform may have been our basic ability to move in response to stimulus, helping us to produce gesture. We know gestural symbols can occur naturally before spoken ones, because gesture precedes language development in children. Infant gestures are important for gaining the attention of a caregiver, increasing the likelihood of an idea or early spoken sound being understood.[378,379] Gesture may have played a similar role in prehistoric communication between adults, providing a springboard for the first examples of something like speech. Today, amongst children and adults, we see often spontaneous gesture supporting speech,[380] through processes that are both conscious and unconscious.

Whichever came first – gesture or speech – there is good reason to think both were used together early on – as they often still are now. Studies of fish show the neural mechanisms for moving pectoral fins (the side fins at the front) share the same networks in the hindbrain as those used for producing sound signals.[381] We might assume our forelimbs evolved from such pectoral fins, and so this coupling of fin movement with sound signals helps explain why vocalisation and forelimb movement can be observed as so synchronised in humans today.[382] The organisation of the human brain also suggests gesture and speech may have arrived together, since producing gesture involves Broca's area[383] – the brain region most famously associated with speech production. As with fish, human language and gesture also produce activity in shared regions of the same underlying neural network.[384]

The arrival of symbols

Many different animals use vocal sounds to warn others of predators, or to attract mates, and many more animals use movement signals to repel aggressors – such as baring their teeth. However, both types of animal communication – gestural and vocal – are emotional responses far removed from a language of abstract symbols. Abstract symbols can retain their meaning irrespective of the context in which they are used. We can use the word "angry" without implying we are angry at this moment, but an animal's anger display is very here and now. Animal communication doesn't seem to transfer to situations without the emotional stimulus that prompted it. A bear being angry is an angry bear – not a bear trying to communicate something about its anger to another bear, such as what made it angry. To know that, the other bear would really need to have been there to see what the fuss is all about.

That said, the first symbols, whether gestural and/or spoken, would have been more closely tied to what was happening in the immediate environment than most human language. They would need to have been. The first symbols would have been rough and ready, and received by minds that were not well prepared for symbols. Whether the first symbols were sounds or gestures, misunderstandings would have been prevalent, and meaning would often have got lost. Gestures are usually closer to concrete common experience than sounds, making it easier for their meaning to be grasped. For example, all stomachs can feel full or empty, so patting the stomach provides a big clue that you are communicating something about food. This makes gesture a more likely candidate for our initial faltering steps in language than speech.[274] Being tied to common contexts would have made the symbols more robust – more likely to be repeated and reinforced, and less likely to be forgotten. This would have helped them survive the poor transmission quality of very primitive language. In the fearful context of an impending predator, the association of a hand wave and a present danger would be easily made – and easily restored in a future situation involving the same type of danger (see emotional memory, Chapter 3).

In captivity, primates with smaller brains than ours can make such associations and use the symbols that are formed to communicate, adding further strength to the "gesture first" hypothesis. One of the most useful gestures is pointing – and although chimpanzees do not use such a gesture in the wild, they can learn to use this gesture from humans when held in captivity. Pointing is a very direct way of communicating the presence of a self-evidently important stimulus (e.g. prey and predators). Its meaning is tied to context but is sufficiently flexible to help communicate many different messages. Pointing can also begin a period of shared attention, potentially supporting more extended communication. There are good reasons, however, why primates other than ourselves don't bother with it. The uncooperative nature of chimpanzee life means that, in the wild, they have little need for pointing and sharing attention. Primates such as marmosets and tamarins are cooperative but have much smaller brains and so less capacity for language generally. If *Homo* was both cooperative and increasingly larger-brained, it would have possessed both the motivation and the accumulating capacity to develop greater use of gestures.

Each advance in the use of symbols potentially improved learning and so improved transfer and distribution of the advance itself across the population, making it a little less likely the new expertise would be lost. For example, if a pointing gesture could successfully start a brief period of shared attention, then any gesture that followed (e.g. patting the stomach to mean food) was more likely to be understood, reinforcing the meaning and memory of both gestures. In this way, symbols would have contributed strongly to a cultural "ratchet effect", discouraging backward slippage and loss of symbols, and so encouraging further cultural progress.

From context-tied communication to abstract symbolism

While context-bound communication was more robust, it was also limited. Pointing, for example, like the sexual and anger displays of animals, requires the here and now for its interpretation.

This tethering to context reduces the usefulness of a symbol. Pointing cannot be used to focus another's attention on a concept that is not actually present. An abstract symbol, on the other hand, is abstract precisely because it is not wholly dependent on context – it can bring to mind a concept that is not related to anything present. Simply learning by association can help achieve this. If repeated use of a gesture causes it to become very strongly associated with the concept, then it may communicate something like its original meaning irrespective of what's happening in the here and now. In this way, the symbol begins to break free – it can be used anywhere, anytime. In principle, if abstraction is about association, it can occur using the same type of unsupervised learning common to other animals – but *Homo*'s generally increased brain power makes this more feasible.

With abstraction, a throwing action can be used to suggest the idea of going hunting, even when no animals worth hunting can be seen in the immediate vicinity. In this example, the idea of hunting is becoming abstracted from reality, i.e. a gesture is bringing hunting to mind in a place where it isn't happening. The spoken word "hunting" takes this process of abstraction one step further, bringing hunting to our mind with a fully abstract symbol that need have no concrete relation to the activity at all.

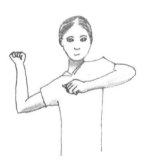

But even the flexibility offered by a primitive throwing gesture starts mushrooming when combined with other primitive gestures. It can, for example, be combined with another symbol and mean the opposite – "let's not go hunting" – instead. This ability to transmit and receive abstract ideas using symbols has been cited as **the** key achievement that elevated *H. sapiens* to top predator. This is largely because abstract symbols encourage reasoning and so the learning of more concepts (see box on p. 109), firing the starting gun for the accumulation of formal knowledge. However, rather than representing a great leap forward in terms of our neurobiology, it most likely arose gradually from the same basic abilities and behaviours we share with other species. Once again, an apparently special human ability is just a natural consequence of being a large-brained primate with a collaborative orientation. That, of course, in no way detracts from the huge significance of abstract symbols for our history. In fact, there would be no history without them!

At some point, a larger gestural vocabulary would have allowed gestures to become sequenced in some sort of structure. When symbols are brought together, the order in which this happens can itself be symbolic. This offers a greater range of messages than the sum of those provided by the symbols on their own. "Man hunts animal" can be perceived as very different in its meaning to "animal hunts man". This ordering, or syntax, is an important dimension of all languages, and it often communicates something about the relation between individual symbols. For example, an established order of activity-target-outcome can begin to indicate causal relationships, like "hunting buffalo gives food", as in the following example:

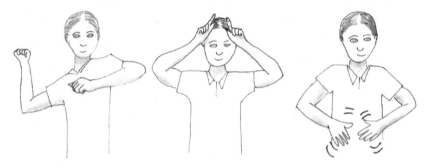

1) Activity: hunting 2) Target: buffalo 3) Outcome: food

Here, if you reverse the sequence . . .

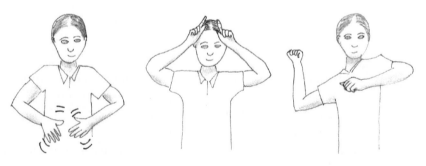

1) Activity: eating 2) Target: buffalo 3) Outcome: hunting

. . . it might mean "eating buffalo makes you go hunting". So, as well as providing more meaning options using the same symbols, syntax can also come to encourage and communicate ideas about cause and effect. The suggestion such complex ideas were being communicated using gesture and syntax alone might be a little fanciful, but it does illustrate how the repertoire of messages can rapidly expand with each symbol acquired.

How do abstract symbols help us learn?

Symbolic language allows for more elaborate and more efficient communication, and so the possibility of faster learning. However, rather than just help us express thought, it can also help generate it. When we turn concrete experience into abstract symbols, it becomes easier to mentally manipulate. In other words, abstract symbols support abstract reasoning.

We can observe the effect of this in the classroom. When a teacher introduces a concept to children using a concrete example, the children find it easier to reason about the concept – but only in respect of this physical example. They can find it difficult to move beyond the particular concrete example provided.

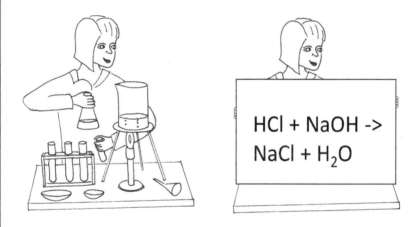

$$HCl + NaOH \rightarrow NaCl + H_2O$$

In contrast, when a concept gets introduced in an abstract way (say, using symbols or drawings), children first find it more difficult to grasp. This is because the children must link their own concrete experience to the abstract representation just to make sense of it. However, once grasped, this abstract representation travels in a way that the concrete example does not. Being shown a concept using an abstract representation like a diagram helps the learner transfer the new knowledge to new contexts.[385] This gives a sense of the intellectual leap made by our species when we first started using abstract symbols, and how this leap empowered us.

This may also suggest something of a dilemma for teachers though – should they be using concrete examples that are easy to grasp or abstract representations that help transfer? Happily, recent investigations confirmed abstract and concrete representations can be complementary.[386] Research shows the potential effectiveness of a "concreteness fading" approach in which the teacher moves gradually from the concrete to the abstract.[387]

Vocalised symbols – the first speech

Amongst early *Homo* communities, learning would have been particularly aided by working together on day-to-day challenges and experiencing life collectively, since this would have encouraged individuals to pay

---

Rhythm and language

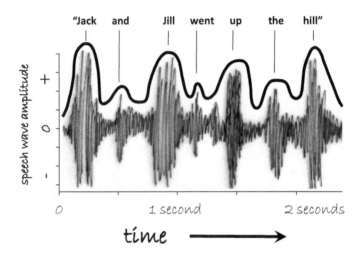

The rhythm of speech helps us break down (or decode) speech into its various parts, and this decoding forms an important basis for learning to understand and produce its written form. Difficulties in reading (dyslexia) often have their developmental roots in difficulty with decoding speech sounds, and here rhythmic training appears to help.[388] The rhythm of speech children hear when they are learning a language assists them in identifying patterns of where the stress is laid, and also how the sounds can be separated into syllables and smaller units.[389] Indeed, although current educational approaches focus greatly on the "phonics" approach, an intervention based on rhythm training appears just as powerful as phonetic training in remediating reading problems.[390] A musical intervention that encourages children to attend closely and accurately to rhythm has also been shown to improve literacy skills.[391] Potentially, such research points to the benefits of singing for literacy and a possible prehistoric role for song in language development. In song, the rhythmic structure of music and language must be locked together. When we sing, we rehearse the important speech rhythm skill that helps us "decode" speech sounds.[389]

---

more attention to each other. This would also have resulted in some types of vocalised sounds being instantly recognisable, more regularly experienced and rehearsed, and so more easily rediscovered and restored through learning. So, for example, verbal imitation of the sounds produced by birds or by producing stone tools may have featured in early spoken communication. These incidental noises have a recognisable rhythm. This makes them easy to imitate and rhythm continues to play an important part in language today (see box opposite). In the early days of language, the link to common non-speech sounds would have helped these sounds survive better than the abstract sounds we use in modern speech.[392] Again, of course, this resemblance would also have meant that these symbols were, at first, more tethered to certain situations. As with gesture, full abstraction would occur when the vocalised sound became so strongly associated with an idea that it could bring this idea into another's mind irrespective of the situation.

The adaptive value of evolving into a teacher

In today's highly social human world, it seems easy to accept the advantages of communicating knowledge. But before language and culture were established, the benefits would not have been so obvious. Evolution is, after all, a competitive process in which individuals better fitted to the environment are more likely to survive and flourish. So how could an individual behaving more like a teacher – and so passing on information more efficiently – have favoured the survival of that individual's genes? At first sight this seems particularly odd, especially if it means the upkeep of extra brain tissue. Teaching tends to be of most benefit to the student. Indeed, if you know something that someone else doesn't, keeping it to yourself can provide a personal advantage!

Teaching requires skilful modification of one's behaviour to aid communication. It must offer some immediate advantage to justify the extra brain capacity required and for this to be passed down generations.[393] The processes involved might include sexual selection. For example, vocal learning from an effective female teacher – perhaps something like a song – might help a male acquire a more complex vocal repertoire. This could then be more favoured by the female whose teaching genes are then more likely to be passed on. Darwin himself suggested our ancestors chiefly used their voices to sing with during courtship,[394] and sexual selection may have helped a musical type of proto-language emerge.[395] This would, however, rely on female *Homo* already having a bias towards males with greater vocal complexity – something that remains to be demonstrated. The other explanation is that better teaching helped transmit information to relatives. Most directly, this would advantage the relatives, but it might indirectly help the teacher's survival through the whole group becoming better informed and more successful. Also, by adding to the survival chances of the other relatives' genes, which would include a lot of the teacher's, it would also add to the survival of the teacher's genes. This is an example of so-called kin selection – when one's genetic relatives get favoured by an individual's adaptation. This favours transmission of many of those genes linked to the individual and that adaptation (even if it doesn't directly help the individual teacher survive and reproduce).

Speech shaping the brain

So far, it appears the genetic brain changes that took place alongside language may not have been directly related to language itself, but more related to greater general flexibility. This is supported by the general, overall increase in brain size. However, two more specific brain changes may also have helped boost our verbal repertoire. In non-human primates, the larynx can produce impressive sounds, but freely willed control over it is limited. Humans benefit from greater connectivity between the larynx and the important motor control centre for vocalisation,[396] supporting greater wilful manipulation of sound. The second key change involves the basal ganglia circuitry (and its connections with the cortex) that we encountered in Chapter 3. Modification here supports improved learning and articulation of speech and language in humans. This modification has been linked to the FOXP2 gene.[397]

A number of genes have been implicated in spoken language development, but perhaps FOXP2 is the best known. This gene is involved with brain and lung development.[398] Its absence in mice causes movement and vocalisation problems, and the ability of songbirds to completely and accurately imitate songs depends upon it. Over the last 500,000 years, a series of mutations occurred in *Homo* FOXP2 which enhanced the connectivity and plasticity of the cortex and basal ganglia circuitry. The process by which FOXP2 expresses itself acquired a human-specific change that was shared by Sapiens, Neanderthals and Denisovans.[354] *H. sapiens*' FOXP2 underwent a final mutation after 260 Kyr, around the time when modern humans first appeared in Africa.[399] Interestingly, the FOXP2 gene differs between Neanderthals and most, but not all, modern humans.[399,400] If this difference was crucial for language, it should be noticeable in the minority of modern Sapiens that lack it, but no research has yet tried to reveal these differences.[401]

FOXP2 controls the expression of many genes involved with our mental abilities[398] and does not just influence language. Nevertheless, it has gained a reputation as a "language gene". This is chiefly due to its involvement in a famous case study of family "KE". A mutation of this gene was linked to problems with language in three generations of this British family, and presence of the disorder could be predicted by presence of the mutation.[402] At first sight, this seems to support the notion that a common language disorder can be caused by a single gene – but this is an idea that is rapidly falling out of favour (see box overleaf).

Language and material culture supporting each other

From ~300 Kyr there is evidence of display behaviour, such as using red ochre – perhaps as body paint. Material culture was also taking forms that do not appear immediately helpful in the harsh day-to-day struggle to survive. These include attractive pebbles, crystals, shells, whale teeth and fossils. But the practical value of these objects may lie in how they helped users to communicate while overcoming some limitations of the more primitive symbols. We have seen, for example, how the concreteness of a gesture can help generate an idea in the mind of an observer. However, that doesn't work when communicating the many ideas that don't have obvious associations with a bodily action (e.g. tree, sun, ant, father). If the concept is not in the immediate vicinity, then pointing won't help either.

Objects of material culture, such as beads, stones and stone tools, had a role to play here. Objects can retain their form better than gestures, which can vary greatly in how they are produced. Many objects can also become easily linked to an activity or context by association. For example, a person's desire to go hunting for meat can be expressed by picking up a meat-hunting tool. The tool is now communicating an idea of hunting for meat – an activity that is not actually occurring in the same time and place as the communication. Not only can material resources support communications beyond the here and now, but they also do not even need the communicator to be present. In this way, material culture was encouraging and supporting the extension of here-and-now primate sociality to something more symbolic.[403] Objects such as stone tools may have been amongst the first human-made symbols, with the symbols of material culture supporting and co-evolving with language using gestures and sound.

Objects have particular potential for encouraging an "education of attention" amongst group members.[404] We saw in Chapter 5 how becoming cultured begins when children are very young, and that "cultured"

Brains, genes and normality . . .

A puzzling question for scientists is why some disorders – such as specific language impairment (SLI) – are still so prevalent, after so many thousands of years of evolution. Children diagnosed with SLI achieve language milestones but much later than normal, often continuing to use simplified syntax and vocabulary as adults. SLI is very common – it affects 3–7% of the population.[405] So, if we think speech was important enough for survival and reproduction to justify its existence in the first place, why didn't natural selection do a better job?

One reason might be that genes predictive of SLI also predict other behaviour that may have been helpful for our ancestors in their prehistoric world. Such an idea has been used to explain today's high prevalence of the traits of Attention Deficit Hyperactivity Syndrome (ADHD). The suggestion is that ADHD genes might once have improved hunting and survival in a hostile environment,[406] only becoming labelled as detrimental in today's agrarian and settled culture. However, it's difficult to offer similar explanations for SLI, if speech ability has sustained its value since it first emerged. Indeed, generally, it seems puzzling that human evolution has not more greatly favoured some particular mental abilities over others.[407]

A more likely explanation may be that SLI and language, along with other complex abilities such as intelligence, are high polygenic – meaning many genes are involved. It is true that you are more likely to develop SLI if one or both of your parents suffer from it, demonstrating that our genes do indeed play an important role in its transmission. However, if our mental abilities (and disorders) arise from the combined effect of many genetic influences interacting with each other and the environment, then individual genes would have little impact on their own.[408,409] This means the natural "selecting out" of unfit genes would be very inefficient, because the fitness contribution of a gene would depend on what it occurred with (i.e. other genes, other environments) – and these would vary from one generation and one individual to the next.[407] Supporters of this multifactorial model point to the increasing numbers of genes found to be related to learning difficulties whose individual effect is small and which also occur amongst the "normal" population.[410] In terms of many learning disorders (including dyslexia, dyscalculia and ADHD), this emphasises the absence of a clear biological dividing line between many outcomes we call "normal" and "abnormal",[410,411] even though these differences may, to a greater and lesser extent, be inherited.

in the most fundamental sense means attending to the attention of others. It can mean, for example, simply looking at where the tool-maker or tool-user is looking when observing them. For our species, this sharing of attention appears intrinsically pleasurable[412] and in existing communities with or without formal education, material culture is still used to achieve this sharing, alongside story-telling, ceremonies and singing.

No special equipment needed?

Current thinking proposes symbolic language and material culture arose naturally when large-brained primates happened upon circumstances that favoured improving their social learning. According to our modern understanding, then, there doesn't seem a need for special equipment. If that's true, one might expect other *Homo* species – or variants on our species – would have left evidence of using symbols too. Interestingly, recent finds do suggest Neanderthals sporadically used red ochre in Northern Europe from around 200–250 Kyr.[413] More strikingly, feathers[414] are also found at many different sites dating from 100 Kyr until Neanderthal extinction at around 30 Kyr.[415] While red ochre can have some practical uses, it is difficult to find any use for feathers that is not purely symbolic. The differences between *H. sapiens* and Neanderthal language abilities, and whether these contributed to their extinction, remain a contested area but there is material culture, genetic and anatomical evidence that suggests Neanderthals possessed some speech capability.[401]

Although no special equipment was needed to get things started, symbols and particularly speech began to change the *Homo* world. Language is still the most powerful tool we have for helping to shape our environment. Even a primitive form of language would have fostered further cooperation and the more efficient transfer of information and skills. This would have resulted in a more social world that, in turn, would have resulted in greater pressure to improve social skills and language. This pressure would increase again, once communication was good enough to ensure practical knowledge could be passed down generations and accumulate over the longer term. The effects of this pressure would have been chiefly to improve language and learning through cultural rather than biological processes. However, if speech and culture were now playing a critical role in the survival and reproduction of individuals, this would also have made a genetic upgrade of our speech-making equipment more likely. By at least 50 Kyr, human fossils show an extension of the vocal tract that allowed *H. sapiens* to speak the vowels [i], [u] and [a]. This extension of the tract makes choking more likely – a dramatic downside that must reflect the original value of such sounds for survival and reproduction.[416]

Creativity and communication within and beyond the group – cultural bursts

Although anatomically modern humans (*H. sapiens*) evolved in Africa 200 Kyr, advances in culture, symbols and tools are hard to detect for another 100,000 years. Evidence of change arrives around 100–80 Kyr[417] but it is often sporadic until 30 Kyr.[418] The discontinuous nature of early cultural progress points to social and cultural processes at work, rather than evolution.[419] Evidence of losses, including whole sets of abilities such as tool-making, clothing and fire, is thought to reflect changes in the environment that disrupted cultures or made the cultural knowledge less useful. Cultural stability may, in part, be due to communication reaching a quality good enough to sustain cultural knowledge across a large enough group to keep it safe from loss. Size of group appears important for accumulating and maintaining new knowledge, and division into smaller groups makes the knowledge held within these groups more vulnerable to being forgotten.[420] Culture suffers when populations fall below a certain threshold and/or when the conventions that help transmit the knowledge get disrupted. For example, over the last 8000 years, the tools used by the Tasmanians lost their complexity once they became isolated from mainland Australia.[421] Pacific island groups have also lost valuable technologies, such as canoes, pottery and the bow and arrow.[422] The explorers Elisha Kane and Isaac Hayes reported how, in the 1820s, an epidemic removed the wise elders of an Inuit group in Greenland. The explorers found the remaining Inuit had no kayaks or bows and arrows, and that their snow houses lacked the usual long heat-saving entryways. They did not know how to hunt caribou or fish in local streams, and could only hunt down seals at certain times of the year. The missing gaps in their knowledge were finally filled when they were visited by another group of Inuit from Baffin Island.[423,424]

If such events explain the losses, what caused the "cultural explosions"? One possibility is that when environmental conditions were good, emerging language allowed a large and diverse set of communities to connect, helping to disperse, stabilise and build their knowledge.[425] The first bursts of cultural sophistication around 45 Kyr may, therefore, simply be a product of demographics. In other words, these were larger populations that were hosting a greater number of particularly skilful social learners. This supported the cultural accumulation and distribution of their knowledge, which was stimulated further by interaction with other such groups.[422,426,427] In short, social connectivity was now linking together the neural networks of individuals to produce a collective processing power that was greater than any one individual's – helping to drive the first flourishes of cultural innovation and creativity. A creative solution to a problem requires making unusual connections with ideas less obviously related to the problem itself, and sometimes we don't need larger networks involving others to help us do this. However, as individuals, we often tend to fixate on the ideas that most feature in our own experience. This usually results in generating the most obvious rather than the more creative of solutions. When our communication skills allow us to share our ideas with others, this makes it easier to avoid fixation, leading to more original ideas than we might otherwise have had on our own (see box below). In this way, larger and more stable social networks would have aided the creation, as well as the communication, of new technologies. When the fit to the environment was good enough to support large, well-connected populations, then more diversity and innovation would have been a natural outcome.

Creativity and sharing ideas

Brain imaging has shed light on the processes which underlie the creative value of sharing ideas.[428] Scientists identified the neural activity associated with creative thinking, and noticed that it involved suppressing activation of a brain region called the angular gyrus. This is a region involved with automatic processing. This suggests participants were trying hard to ignore their automatic and obvious solutions when trying to be creative. The scientists then compared what happened when, before expressing their ideas, participants either "incubated" these ideas or reflected on the ideas of others. Reflecting on the ideas of others caused the participants to find more original responses, and it led to less deactivation of the angular gyrus – suggesting participants found it easier to avoid fixating on the obvious. If sharing of ideas means we are less likely to fixate, this helps explain how the means to communicate between groups with different cultures, technologies and ideas can lead naturally to greater creativity.

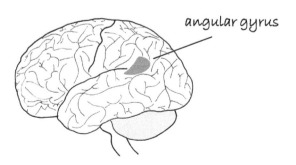

angular gyrus

Every step forward in cultural progress would have helped increase the resistance to slippage and loss of knowledge in the face of natural disaster, but none were sufficient to guarantee a clear sense of cultural progress for many thousands of years. From around 20 Kyr we begin to see *continuous* accumulation of objects which are not purely functional. The meaning and value of such objects had stabilised – and so the culture which was communicating this meaning must have too. This suggests a step change in how knowledge was being transmitted and the existence of a robust language that could be passed down through time. The information network had grown from one-to-one grooming activities, to verbal and gestural communications that could sustain larger social groups, to a fully symbolic and stable spoken language enabling communication within and between large populations. Depending on the ebb and flow of culture, it was possible for individuals to communicate with and learn from those they had never met, and with whom they shared no living space or close family. Learning was now being supported by a shared set of symbols whose meaning was being culturally inherited across generations.

7

THE ARRIVAL OF NUMERACY

E ARE FAST APPROACHING the arrival of numeracy and literacy in our history of the learning brain. These skills may have revolutionised our culture but they are recent and their distribution in the human population has been patchy. That tends to suggest they didn't involve changes in our genetic make-up. If true, that means our brain is now "special enough" for these things to emerge through learning, rather than evolution. So how special is that?

What's so special about the human brain?

The human brain is often celebrated as amazing, but is it much more amazing than the brain of other animals? To make the case, scientists have used a range of measures to claim human superiority. There are some measures, however, that we just cannot compete on. The weight of our brain is several times smaller than that of African and Asian elephants[429] and several different types of whale.[430,431] Our brains do, just, have the largest weight of cortex as a percentage of the whole brain (around 76%). This might be important, because the cortex has been associated more with reasoning than regions such as the cerebellum, which is more about coordinating actions and senses. However, chimpanzees,[431,432] horses and short-finned whales[433–438] achieve 73%, 75% and 73%, respectively, so our 76% hardly matches the status we give our mental abilities.

More sophisticated measures have also been used. These include accounting for the absolute size of an animal, in attempts to show that the human brain scales up altogether differently. When brain size is mapped against body size, a general "power law" emerges. The extent to which an animal departs from this trend is termed the *encephalisation quotient* (EQ). The EQ might suggest extra neural processing beyond what's needed to monitor and coordinate a larger body. For this reason, EQ has been used to represent animal intelligence instead of brain size, and we do well on this scale. The human brain has around a seven times greater brain-to-body mass ratio than expected for a mammal, and threefold greater than expected even for a primate. However, a study of the relation between EQ and cognitive ability across non-human primates shows EQ is, after all, not a good predictor of intelligence.[234]

The number of neurons may represent a better indicator of basic processing power. As we saw in Chapter 4, primates boast a very efficient approach to packing in neurons compared with other mammals.[439–441] The human brain follows the same primate packing rule and we have the expected number of neurons for a primate brain of our size.[167] So, we may not have the biggest brain but we have the biggest primate brain and that's good news: it results in us having the largest number of neurons of all animals. We don't have the 100 billion neurons the popular press often refers to, but we do have an estimated 86 billion neurons compared with, for example, a gorilla's 33 billion neurons.

We are fortunate in having so many neurons but, beyond that, we cannot say the human brain is biologically extraordinary compared with other species.[441] If our chief advantage arises from our enlarged brain being a primate brain, then this advantage would not have been unique to *Homo sapiens*. The fossilised skulls of other, extinct *Homo* primates provide a reasonable estimate of the size of the brain they protected.[442] Applying the primate neuron-packing rule to the fossil record suggests archaic *Homo* members such as *heidelbergensis* and *neanderthalensis* reached capacities of 76–90 billion neurons, well within the range of modern humans.[443]

Counting neurons also raises doubts about whether the size of cortex to cerebellum indicates a bias towards higher-order reasoning. Across orders of mammals, it seems that, even when the cortex dominates brain volume, the ratio of neurons in the cortex to those in the cerebellum remains roughly the same. It's just the way neurons are packed that makes the volume of cortex to cerebellum expand across evolutionary time.[444]

In short, the simple answer to what's most special about our own brain is just that, at the moment, we have the largest *primate* brain on the planet. While that may deflate our sense of being extraordinary, it reminds us how we are part of the web of life and should be respectful of that web. As well as protecting it, we should also allow it to teach us about ourselves. Also, everything that science is learning about the brain, almost irrespective of which animal we are talking about, has only added to our impression of its general complexity. So, in this sense, we have never had greater reason to be wowed by brain sophistication; we just shouldn't get too hung up on the idea that our brain is particularly more amazing than any other animal's.

But now . . . accepting that the arrival of numeracy and literacy did not involve some evolutionary leap presents a clear challenge for our story. We need an explanation of how numeracy and literacy arose from a brain not evolved to do these things. How, in a world without written numbers and words, could these skills could have been invented and transmitted culturally?

The shifting sands of culture

Genes are stable and sexual reproduction ensures mostly faithful transmission across generations. On the other hand, cultural transmission of an ability is potentially much more fragile. That means it was easy for communities and groups within our species to occasionally lose the cultural tools of calculation and writing, particularly when they were first emerging. It took thousands of years for them to be represented in widely accessible material forms (e.g. books) that could ensure they were faithfully passed down. So, it would be wrong to assume these skills arrived at a single moment and were continuously accumulated and dispersed. Instead, they would have been created, lost and rediscovered within prehistoric groups and communities many times over – as environmental and cultural histories unfolded. They had to naturally emerge many times in prehistory, from a mental "platform" unadapted for these specific purposes – and which remains unadapted for these purposes today.

That means we can learn much about the prehistoric arrival of number abilities by studying how we learn them now. When we see learners first encounter number, we are watching processes at play that come from a much older evolutionary history than the Stone Age. Our formal maths arises from ancient abilities to automatically sense quantity – abilities shared with other vertebrates but aided, in our case, by a primate sociality and spoken language.

Subitising – an ancient number sense good for lunch

The word "subitising" comes from the Latin word *subitus* – meaning "sudden". If we see a set of four objects or fewer, we can experience a feeling of just "suddenly knowing" how many items there are. For example, when you look at the following sets of dots, you can immediately choose the greater set in each pair – you don't have to stop and count:

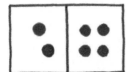 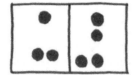 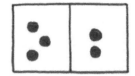

We share this ability with many mammals,[445–448] birds[449,450] and even fish.[451,452] Its evolution is thought to have been driven by the need to pursue prey efficiently, allowing animals to track up to around four travelling lunches in parallel, even if these were moving and occasionally out of sight.[453]

Subitising develops automatically so it can be quite simple for a child to start labelling small quantities as "1", "2", "3" or "4" in spoken language. They just have to map names to these quantities through association, as they hear others around them using the correct number word in contexts involving that quantity. This "direct mapping" means children can begin to learn how many objects there are without being able to formally count them. This is provided, of course, the numbers are in their subitising range – and this range develops with age. At around two years old, children are "one-knowers", i.e. they can give you one object if you ask for it. Requests for any quantity larger than one (two, three, etc.) will result in you receiving a random number of objects (but more than one). After another 6–9 months, they can deliver "one", "two" or "more" objects, before later becoming "three-knowers".

Subitising bootstraps counting

But that would be the end of the line using this approach alone. Direct mapping can't help you with larger numbers since the subitising range, even in adults, is limited to around four. However, at the same time, the novice counter will have been learning a longer number sequence (e.g. 1 to 10) as they hear it repeated around them, even though they don't yet grasp its full meaning. Often children are heard reciting this sequence as though it were a rhyme or song, but they are still grabbing an apparently random number of objects when asked for more than about four.

Armed with the counting sequence and an awareness of the meaning of its first few numbers, children must now make an all-important link: there is an analogy between the position of a certain number in the counting sequence and the quantity of a set of objects. In other words, to count to five and beyond, children must grasp the cardinality principle: *the last number-word used in the counting sequence indicates the number of items in the set.* In this way, their association of the smaller number-words with quantities they can already subitise will "bootstrap"[i] their meaning of the number-words for the larger quantities. They can now map symbols (i.e. words) to quantities.

Counting is cultural

The steps that extend our animal senses into a formal concept of number are challenging for learners. Fortunately, in communities that use number, children have parents, peers and teachers who, consciously or otherwise, can support their learning of counting. These others often encourage children to speak number words in their subitising range ("1", "2", "3") when looking at objects of the right quantity, to rehearse the counting sequence, and to speak this sequence while each new object in a set of such objects is pointed to once. Such talk makes it more likely that the all-important analogy will be made, and the cardinality rule will be grasped and memorised. This use of language to support knowledge "under construction" is another example of the *scaffolding* we came across in Chapter 5.

The cultural nature of number is highlighted when the scaffolding language influences how the cardinality rule is learnt. This is because different languages represent quantity in slightly different ways. In English, for example, unlike Japanese and Chinese, you have to signal whether a word is singular or plural, saying "three cups" rather than "three cup". This helps explain why English children grasp the concept of "one" more quickly than Japanese and Chinese children.[454,455] Other languages have three ways to mark a noun's number so, in Slovenian, "button" can occur as one (*gumb*), two (*gumba*) or the plural (*gumbi*), and this helps explain why Slovenian children learn the meaning of "two" more quickly than English children.[456] The way language is used around a child is known to influence their numeracy and, when children's parents talk about the number of objects around them, children learn more quickly about numbers.[457–459] Understanding numbers is very much about interaction with others, rather than a child's independent reflection. Without others providing scaffolding, even learning to count beyond four or five must be very challenging.

But to understand the prehistoric origins of mathematics, that is exactly what we have to imagine. We must think of the straightforward mapping of one, two and three to spoken words and then the cardinality principle emerging in a world where no such scaffolding existed, at least in the social and cultural sense. In that world, other forms of scaffolding may have been critical in the discovery and frequent rediscovery of counting. What could these other forms of scaffolding have been?

Fingers and numbers

In Chapter 6, we saw how creating gestures would have helped spoken language develop in prehistory and may even have preceded it. Our understanding of maths and its symbols may also have some important roots in the form and actions of our body. Our hands, and more specifically our fingers, can provide a simple symbolic representation of number, as a set of (up to) 10 objects that are always available. Expressing numbers with fingers provides a convenient and visual way to support thinking and communicating about number to others.

Talking number with fingers would have been easiest with numbers in the subitising range up to around four, but it is easy to imagine how the fifth finger could then have become involved. Social interactions involving finger talk, as often occur today, may have greatly helped bootstrap the connection between the number sequence and the number of objects. When the cardinality principle emerged, the remaining fingers were standing by to help larger numbers up to 10 be understood, represented and communicated across generations.

All this suggests a strong association between our primitive sense of quantity and our hands, and fingers are persistently and prevalently used for counting across cultures despite the increased availability of digital technologies.[460–463] Stock exchange traders, for example, still communicate to each other with fingers, although using a single hand, while the other is usually grasping a more modern form of communication:

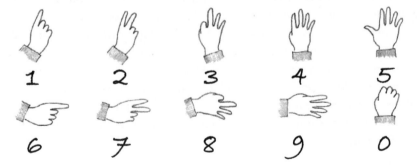

Biological evidence points to a long-lasting prehistoric connection between fingers and numbers. In the human brain, being asked to rapidly estimate a quantity activates certain regions in the parietal lobe.[464–470] These regions also activate during reaching, pointing and grasping movements and even when passively watching graspable objects such as tools.[471] When we make small number judgements, the signals to the muscles of our right hand activate. Our number abilities show strange interference effects related to grasping. Our ability to count is disrupted by hand movements unrelated to counting,[472] while related hand movements can support counting and simple arithmetic.[473,474]

This close relationship between fingers and number may have educational implications, with one study showing that simply making children more aware of their fingers can improve the development of their early number skills[475] – see box below.

Finger controversy

An intervention study has shown simply getting to know your fingers (finger gnosis) might improve young children's numerical ability. This is contrary to the recommendations of many mathematics educators to discourage finger counting and so foster more "in the head" calculation. Researchers[475] assessed new arrivals at three Belgian primary schools for finger gnosis and formed three groups. The first group comprised children who performed very well in their finger gnosis. The first interesting finding was that these children had better counting skills. The rest of the children were assigned to a control group or a group that followed a finger gnosis training programme for two half-hour sessions per week over eight weeks. Training consisted of games played with coloured stickers on each fingernail. For example, in one game the children followed each coloured pathway in a maze with the correspondingly coloured finger.

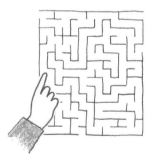

After the training period, the children who had received the training in finger gnosis performed significantly better at quantification tasks and the processing of written numbers. These positive results have not resolved the debate between neuroscientists and mathematics educators regarding the role of fingers.[476]

The cardinality principle itself is a cultural invention, and does not exist amongst communities for whom numbers beyond four have little everyday usefulness. The extent to which learning this principle exploited an innate quantity-finger link is not known but, given its role in communication, this link is inevitably influenced by social and cultural forces. Children's early tendency to use their fingers for numbers shows in an additional delay when counting beyond the maximum number one hand is used for. This delay can be observed in adults and varies according to the cultural traditions of how fingers/hands are used, being six in Germany and nine in China.[470]

Hold that thought . . .

Holding up a number of fingers can also help store information while our attention moves elsewhere for a moment (provided, of course, you keep the fingers where they are). This relieves our working memory (our ability to hold information in our conscious attention – see p. 51). This can be helpful because thoughts about the quantity of objects often need to occur with thoughts about their features – such as when counting the number of fruit that are edible. Fingers can keep the tally while the quality of each fruit is considered. Fingers can compensate for life's distractions, because they help *externalise* our thoughts about quantity, moving from an internal effortful representation in our brain to something which exists outside of us, requiring little or no effort to maintain it.

Representing quantity using the body also opened up possibilities for "chunking" information. This is a common strategy for coping with our limited working memory. For example, as an Englishman who already knows the date 1066 (when the French invaded), it would be easy for me to be dictated someone's telephone number in one go, if it was 1231066. This is because 1066 represents a single chunk of information in my mind, and the digits 123 are already "chunked" as the first three digits in the counting sequence. That means that, really, I only have to remember two pieces of information (counting, French invasion). The fact that we have five fingers on each hand, and we have one pair of hands with 10 fingers in total, also helps "chunk" these units together conceptually. So, although a novice to counting may feel daunted by the thought of comparing numbers as large as 60 and 80, the difference between these numbers is easier to think about as the difference between six and eight pairs of hands. We can even calculate this difference using fingers, if each finger represents a pair of hands (answer = two fingers, which really represents two pairs of hands of fingers, or 20). The difference between 65 and 87 is more difficult, of course. However, as we shall see, we share quantity skills beyond just subitising with other animals – including skills that can provide a little extra support for dealing with larger quantities.

The approximate number system

Another type of ancient ability comes into play when we start grappling with large numbers. Although we cannot automatically identify quantities beyond our subitising range exactly, we can automatically *estimate* them. Like other animals, we sense the size of these larger quantities. This sense of quantity is sometimes called numerosity and we experience it as we do other types of physical experience, such as light intensity, the loudness of a sound or the weight of an object. Similar rules apply governing how easy or difficult we find detecting difference. One of these rules is called the distance effect. For example, it can be easy to determine if there is a difference when glancing (without counting) at two piles of 30 and 20 apples (below left). This becomes more difficult as the distance, or difference, between the two quantities decreases. Sensing the difference between 30 and 29 apples is quite tricky (below right):

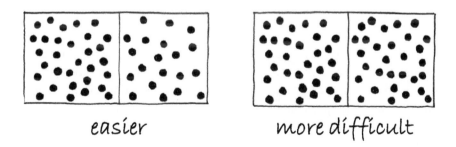

easier   more difficult

We also find it easier when the large:small ratio between the two numbers is higher. This is called the ratio effect. So, although the distance is the same, it is easier to detect the difference when we see 12 and 8 apples (with a ratio of 6:4, on the left), than when we see 20 and 16 apples (with a ratio of 5:4, on the right):

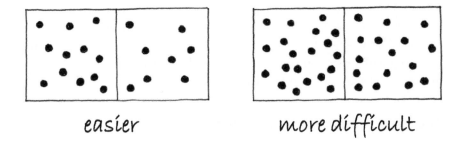

easier   more difficult

Our approximate sense of number, including these distance and ratio effects, exists in other animals such as rodents. This suggests our intuitive and noisy "mental number line" evolved over deep time, well before the advent of our own species.

Education straightens out our number line

When pre-school children are asked to mark numbers on a line with 1 at one end and 10 at the other, the bigger numbers tend to get bunched up towards the end:

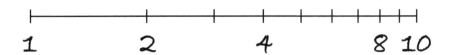

1   2   4   8 10

Measurements of how neurons fire in the primate brain suggest this is the natural "logarithmic" scale we should expect from our brain – before, that is, it has been trained by education. This scale echoes our sensory experience, because it suggests the significance of an increase or decrease is relative to where you start from. So, a decrease from four to two is similar to a decrease from eight to four, but not eight to six. On a socially intimate level, where you want take into account personal circumstances, this can make sense. If you gave me two of your four oranges yesterday, perhaps I should be prepared to share four of my eight oranges today. We are, after all, both giving up half of what we have. In this context, representing quantities in terms of our own personal "sense" of them feels appropriate.

Early number education, on the other hand, emphasises the importance of the linear scale and absolute values, where numbers are equally spaced out on the line:

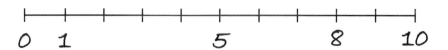

In their lessons, children constantly rehearse the idea that the difference between two and four is the same as between four and six. Here, balance means an orange for an orange. This is important for developing an idea of quantity which is abstract, and not rooted in a personal context. This approach to number allows communication of quantity across large populations. As we learn about numbers and their abstract relation to each other, our representation of them on the number line becomes more precise[477–479] and their spacing on the number line becomes more linear.[480,481] This change to a linear fit is associated with improved maths achievement,[481,482] emphasising the importance of this representation for future ability to deal abstractly with number. Practice using a linear number line has been shown to improve children's ability to correctly solve mathematical problems (see box overleaf).

Animal intuitions help guide our maths

It's very debatable whether our noisy number line helps young children acquire the cardinality principle and so learn to count. It certainly cannot substitute for our abilities using number symbols, which appear more important for success.[483,484] However, our number line can provide some additional help. An automatic sense of magnitude provides a rapid guide and check when number procedures are new and error-prone, so problems with this ability can be expected to impact on the learning of maths. At the beginning of school, children who can only detect the largest distances between quantities tend to end up with poorer maths scores at the end of their first year.[485] An ability to sense magnitude helps us acquire many formal maths skills including, for example, calculations involving fractions.[486] Children learn at around 8–9 years old that ⁶⁄₉ can be simplified as ⅔ and the formal way to do this is to divide the top and the bottom by three (a common factor of six and nine). A common mistake for the novice is to *subtract* a common factor from the top and bottom number instead of dividing into them. This would produce ³⁄₆, but most children can detect (without counting) that getting three pieces of a chocolate bar that comes as six parts is not as good as getting six pieces when the chocolate bar comes as nine parts.

The importance of a linear number line for maths understanding

Children diagnosed with developmental dyscalculia find it particularly difficult to think about and remember mathematical knowledge and to carry out the procedures required for calculations.[487] More fundamentally, these children also have problems mentally representing numbers, and neuro-imaging evidence suggests functional and structural differences in parietal brain regions associated with the mental number line.[435]

A neuroimaging study has shown how training aimed at improving the representation of numbers in dyscalculic children had beneficial effects both on mathematical performance and brain function related to number representation.[488] The study involved children training up their mental number line using a computer game. Children learned to respond to number-related questions by moving a joystick to land a spaceship on the point on a number line that corresponded to their answer.

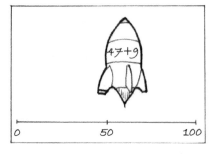

Our ability to sense magnitude helps us rapidly determine the difference between simple ratios, helping to guide our attempts to rehearse a formal approach until these formal processes are secure.

Rehearsal and learning progress

Even with help from our fingers, our working memory is always taxed when we're learning new ways of dealing with a lot of information. When we're learning how to tackle a new process involving numbers, we must think about the numbers themselves, which stage we have reached in the process and what this stage involves. How well we cope with this extra burden on our working memory (i.e. our working memory capacity) will

After training, children with and without dyscalculia improved their arithmetic ability. Analysis of data from both groups showed reduced activation (suggesting greater processing efficiency) in a range of brain regions (shown in white) when performing a number line task:

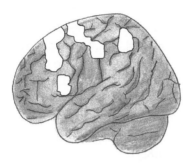

Improvements in both ability and brain activity were, however, greater for the dyscalculic group. Studies such as this, which focus both on problematic learner differences and their remediation, are helpful and relevant to education. First, they provide insight into the biology of individual differences which, when together with educational expertise, may form the basis of more effective teaching approaches. More generally, they show the plasticity of the brain and how brain function can be improved by students practising well-designed tasks. Learning disorders may be associated with distinct neurological differences, but such differences can be responsive to appropriate teaching and learning environments. This simple fact may be helpful in fostering the types of positive teacher attitudes linked to better outcomes for students diagnosed with learning disorders.[489]

influence how quickly we can learn. Since our working memory capacity is quite limited (about seven items – plus or minus two), it can be thought of as a learning bottle-neck. How can we move on to even more complex tasks and processes if we are already using all our working memory capacity?

Practising tasks, including maths tasks, can go a long way towards solving this problem. When we start off with a new task, we must think consciously about what to do with the numbers, how to order and rearrange them, and keep track of where we are in this new process. However, as we practise, some of this becomes more automatic. When a child is first learning to add two and three, they will use some counting procedure, perhaps first with fingers and then without. Eventually, however, they will learn what 2 + 3 is and simply retrieve the answer automatically from memory.

Going back to our more complex example of simplifying fractions, a good amount of practice can also help this become a more automatic process. A well-rehearsed student who sees ⁹⁄₆ may almost immediately recognise the possibility of top and bottom numbers having common factors, and just "know" there is a possibility that it can be reduced to something much simpler. This shift from conscious to more automatic processes is reflected in a shift in brain activity, as demonstrated in a study of adults learning complex multiplication.[490] The brains of these adults were scanned while attempting complex multiplication, before and after a training programme in which they rehearsed this type of maths task many times. A shift in activity was seen away from frontal regions associated with working memory towards posterior regions (more towards the back of the brain) that are associated with more automatic processing. This unburdening of working memory with practice is important, because it frees up the working memory resources needed for further learning to occur. Practice, therefore, does not just perfect our performance but also paves the way for us to learn more.

Technology for information processing – material artefacts that support brain function

A lot can be achieved with fingers and practice, but the ability to produce material culture soon offered new and more powerful methods to *externalise* quantities and the processes that involve them. These technologies helped free up mental resources for reasoning and supported our long-term memory with a physical record that could last over years. In a Stone-Age environment, an obvious way to move beyond fingers was to employ whatever sticks and stones were lying around to represent quantity. These, of course, would be difficult to identify now as archaeological evidence. The oldest identified objects with potential for scaffolding number are beads. The use of beads extends back almost 100,000 years.[491] Amongst these, the small, blue shells with punched holes found in the Blombos Cave in South Africa are the earliest good candidates for the job:[492]

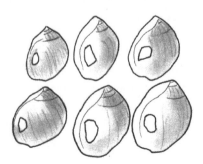

Dated to 77 Kyr, the holes show traces of wear that indicate they were strung, allowing them to be moved along and so, potentially, provide a counting technology. Beads, of course, have multiple uses that include self-decoration, so finding a set of beads is hardly archaeological proof of accounting. However, the properties of beads on a string are notably helpful for grasping concepts of number. They maintain their sequence, as do numbers, and it only requires the attachment of an individual name to each bead for an accounting technology to emerge. This makes them eminently helpful as a physical aid for counting, and they become common at sites dating from around 30 Kyr.[493,494]

While beads and natural objects do not leave convincing traces of number technology, a tool for recording and applying astronomical data provides clearer evidence. As early as 28,000 years ago, a member of our species carved scratches on a small piece of reindeer bone near Sergeac, France and produced the so-called Abri Blanchard artefact.[495] These marks appear to represent the phases and movements of the moon:[496]

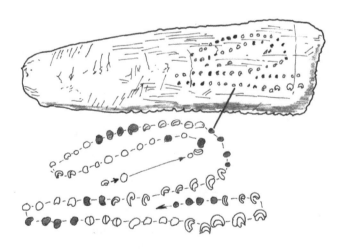

This suggests material culture was being used to augment our brain power in respect of working memory (i.e. to support reasoning when making predictions) and our long-term memory (e.g. helping us to recall specific astronomical events). Often our emerging ideas are somewhat rudimentary, and making them explicit can help clarify them. This artefact would have supported its creator in making his/her ideas more fully formed and to apply them in making astronomical predictions. It also provided a tangible means by which they could be shared, even over generations.[497]

Other artefacts appear more suited to solving problems that were purely numerical, such as the Tossa de la Roca plaque from around 14 Kyr:[498]

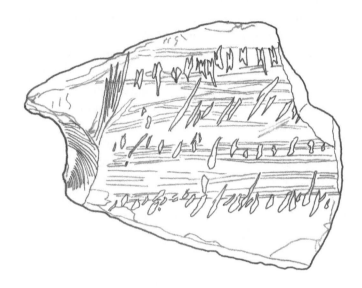

This plaque shows marks engraved using different tools at different times. Someone appears to be keeping track of something, and they were using technology to process quantities that were well beyond their subitising range.[499]

Settling down

Although we know that the mental and material resources for numbers existed during the Stone Age, we should not assume that maths knowledge always steadily accumulated. A diversity of number systems would have existed that differed widely in their complexity, with different approaches being rediscovered and lost many times over.[500] As amongst hunter-gatherers today, the level of complexity of these systems would have reflected the demands of the culture, e.g. what customs were shared, what types of food resource were available and what practices were used to harvest them. Also, depending on the lifestyle, formal counting might often have not been useful enough to bother with at all.

Around 10 Kyr we see the dawn of the Neolithic or "new Stone Age". This was the age that was to begin with agriculture and end with the widespread use of metal tools. It began in the Fertile Crescent – a relatively moist and fertile crescent-shaped region in the otherwise arid environment of Western Asia, the Nile Valley and Nile Delta:

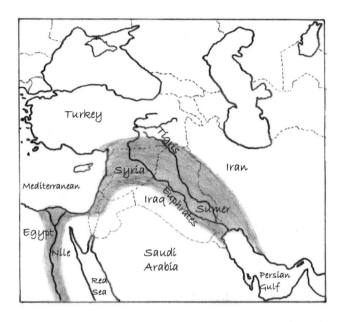

Previously, climate fluctuations during the last Ice Age had made agriculture all but impossible but, when this ended about 11.6 Kyr, farming offered a competitive advantage. Around this time, radio carbon dating of finds in Galilee (Israel) shows intensive farming of the faba bean when water was plentiful. It continued into the next millennium under dryer conditions, as local farmers learnt to select seeds that could germinate in these drier conditions.[501] However, climate alone does not explain the changing pattern of agriculture very well,[502] and culture may have played a critical role. Changes in both climate and society are likely to have driven the change of lifestyle from hunter-gatherer to farming. This is a transition that has never been completed. Until the European expansion of the nineteenth century, 20% of the world's population were still hunter-gatherers, attesting to strong sociocultural factors influencing the spread of farming, with only a slow and shifting development of the more complex social organisation required.[503] This social organisation sustained larger populations and involved people living in large villages that were inhabited all year round. Ultimately this organisation was to support commerce that would help transform the economic, social and technological landscape. We find evidence of trade and exchange between regions in the shell, greenstone, malachite and bitumen discovered in the earliest agricultural settlements of the Fertile Crescent.[504] In some important respects, the fuller consequences of Sapiens flexibility were now becoming apparent.

That said, larger populations and a trend towards economy of scale resulted in greater demand for individuals and individual communities to use their general flexibility to specialise. This tendency to specialisation, and a tethering to the land, would have been a key driver of trade for those settling to a farming lifestyle. Farm produce needed exchanging for the minerals and physical resources required to survive, and numeracy beyond the subitising range would have been a real bonus when bartering.

When the Sumerians settled to agrarian culture in the valley of the Tigris and Euphrates Rivers around 8000 to 7500 BC, they left behind a variety of clay geometric shapes (cones, spheres, disks, cylinders, etc.). These are thought to have been used as tokens – providing a flexible way to support externalising number.[505] These so-called "plain" tokens have simple geometric forms with a smooth surface and no markings, but they possess a variety of shapes including spheres, disks, cones, tetrahedrons and cylinders. These shapes may not be greatly significant, perhaps reflecting the easiest shape to create from the original stone used to produce each one. On the other hand, they may have denoted different values, providing a formal way of "chunking" quantities of smaller units into a range of larger ones, enabling exact manipulation of large quantities.

Plain tokens also made their appearance alongside agriculture. The earliest ones are found amongst villages of round huts that are typical of the hunter-gatherer-to-farmer transition. While trading amongst hunter-gatherers is often revealed by the presence of obsidian, early finds of tokens coincide with large increases in cereal pollen in the soil and other evidence for cultivation and hoarding of grain. This suggests that the tokens were being used for the planning of subsistence over the year,[506] and that some type of record of observations was being kept, perhaps for others to be able to understand. Debate continues as to how the symbolism of these tokens should be interpreted, but some sort of asynchronous communication appears to have arrived. Accountancy, it would seem, was the sign that prehistory was about to end. A new age of written history, in which we record events in detail for others to read, was about to begin.

Note

i   "Bootstrap" is a phrase that scientists have borrowed from the expression "pull yourself up by your bootstraps", implying a self-starting process that requires no extra assistance.

8

THE EMERGENCE OF THE WRITTEN WORD

L IKE NUMBER, WRITING WAS not a unique event that spread outward
like an irreversible wave of progress. Instead, the creation of writing appears to be a human response to life getting complicated,
and it was invented and re-invented many times over.[507] The first
examples are found in the Fertile Crescent from around 4000 BC, when we
find communities beginning to urbanise, expand and collect together as part
of the Sumerian temple institution – an early form of state. The city-state of
Uruk is perhaps the earliest example of writing being created. Towards the
end of Uruk's prominence, around 3500–3300 BC, its administrators were
communicating and recording in several different ways: through tokens, seals
and simple pictures expressed on tablets. The old clay tokens used for expressing numbers made an appearance in two-dimensional form in this archaic
Uruk tablet – which may represent the oldest stage of Sumerian writing:[508]

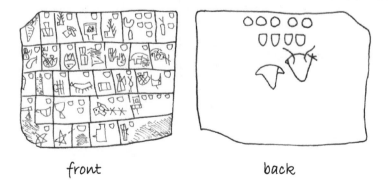

front   back

On the front of the tablet, cone tokens occur with a variety of other signs divided into compartments, providing the appearance of a ledger. On the back of the tablet a cow's head and a bull's head appear under a line of spheres (each representing a group of units – possibly 10) and a line of cones representing one unit each.

Most of the pictures used for writing during this period were quite naturalistic, but some were already becoming more symbolic. For example, the sign for a sheep was simply ⊕. Within a few hundred years, symbols were laid on their backs, naturalistic features were being left out and curved lines were straightened and set to particular angles.[508] The new lines were being created by pressing a cut reed into clay, producing the familiar wedge-shapes of cuneiform script:

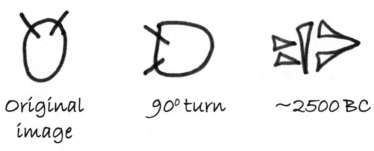

Original   90° turn   ~2500 BC
image

Accountancy ledgers were the first writings and they soon tell us more detail about the world than simply quantity. They describe something about who is doing the transaction. Some early archaic texts, for example, record the accounts of a temple dedicated to the goddess of love (Inanna), where goods were being collected and redistributed:

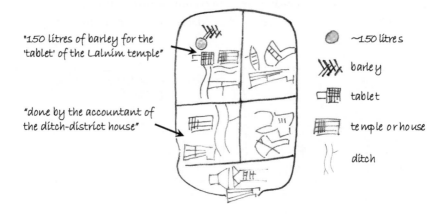

"150 litres of barley for the 'tablet' of the Lalním temple"

"done by the accountant of the ditch-district house"

⬤ ~150 litres

barley

tablet

temple or house

ditch

These accounts supported the temple's business, including the collection of taxes which, for any state, is a critical process. The accounts show the impressive number skills that the Sumerians were developing, with 60 different symbols for expressing quantities in several different number systems (or "bases"). Beyond the use of number, the written contents of the tablets might not sound so inspiring, e.g. "150 litres of barley (~93 kg) for the tablet of the Lalnim Temple" or "done by the accountant of the ditch-district house",[509] but these are the first signs of a written history emerging.

This primitive writing consisted almost entirely of *logograms*, so each symbol represented a whole word or phrase. This was a very different approach to using phonograms to represent speech sounds, such as "ck" to represent the sound /k/ in "back", or "oy" to represent /oi/ as in "toy". A purely logographic language is very limited and no established language, ancient or modern, has ever restricted itself entirely to logograms. The symbols in Ancient Egyptian, for example, can sometimes refer to the sounds of the consonants in the concept's name rather than the concept, and modern Chinese symbols contain elements that provide clues as to the pronunciation.

Occasionally, the accountants had to refer to something or someone for which no picture symbol existed. To get around this, the early writers found they could use existing symbols for things that sounded like parts of the word they wanted to write. This is the so-called rebus principle (rebus meaning "by things" in Latin). In English, for example, the word "treaty" could be represented by a picture of a tree and cup of tea: "tree-tea". In this way, the principle converts pictures into phonograms, which refer to speech sounds. The rebus principle was particularly helpful for communicating proper names. This principle can be found only very occasionally amongst the earliest writings from Mesopotamia, but within a few hundred years we see symbols commonly used to represent sounds. The reader was now being regularly required to decode the symbols into the spoken sound in order to grasp the concept. One of the clearest early examples of a written speech sound comes from Sumerian writings after the decline of Uruk, during the Jemdet Nasr period (3100–2900 BC). Here, in this record of income and redistribution for a Sumerian temple, the writer has taken advantage of the fact that the sound (gi) for "reed" and for the verb "reimburse" in Sumerian are similar.[508] In the top left-hand corner, they have expressed reimbursement in writing using the symbol for a reed:[510]

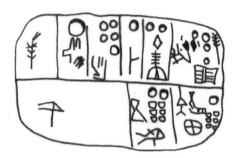

The Sumerians extended the power of their language to express meaning by including more phonetic elements, and it gradually became more recognisable as the written representation of a spoken language. Over the next few hundred years, Akkadian culture displaced Sumerian but the Akkadians adapted the Sumerian writing system to express their own language. No doubt bolstered by having a concrete written form, the language family to which Akkadian belongs (Semitic) has flourished into the present day.

All writing in the world does not have its roots in Sumeria, however. It has also emerged elsewhere in response to other varieties of complex society. The first writings in China, on turtle shells and the shoulder-blades of oxen, tackled social complexity. These were used to express divine responses to queries at the Shang court.[511] The first Maya writing tackled the intricacies of how religious and cultural notions could be intertwined in a sophisticated calendar. This was an issue with immense significance for such a highly ordered society. The general pattern of commerce driving numeracy, with written literacy arriving sometime after, has been repeated elsewhere. Caral was the first urban community in the New World (Peru) and here we find evidence of material scaffolding of numeracy in the form of a stone engraving of a "khipu". Dating from around 4.5 Kyr,[512] the khipu is a knotted-string device thought to have been used well into the last millennium by the Incas for accountancy and communication:[513,514]

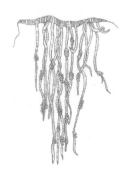

Writing in these parts was not to arrive for another few thousand years, but the early city-dwellers at Caral thrived by growing cotton for the fishing nets of those living many miles away on the coast. The immediate needs of settled existence appear to have made trading and, therefore, recording numbers a more urgent and useful innovation than other types of writing.

We can assume that advances in symbolism (such as that used for trade) helped change many aspects of lifestyle, such as diet. Changes related to diet and disease can easily help bring about genetic changes in a population. For example, symbolic communication occurred alongside dairy farming in Europe and helped it emerge and flourish. Amongst pastoral populations, this is thought to have created selection pressures that favoured the gene variant (or *allele*) for absorbing lactose. However, beyond these indirect effects, we can be fairly confident that the advent of written language did not arrive with any genetic adaptation. This is because it began so late in the story of the brain's evolution and was, until the last hundred years, meaningless to the vast majority of the world's population. As with numeracy, evolution helps us understand reading and writing by drawing attention to how they must be continuously arising from abilities we evolved to do other things.

Forms of writing and brain development

Our brains evolved to encounter a wide range of "expected" environmental influences at infancy that did not include print. Sensitive periods exist during this early development when primary functions, such as our hearing and vision, use these encounters to "tune" themselves. By the time an individual's brain begins to read, write and count, some of the general-purpose plasticity of the cortex has been reduced and some tuning is already complete. This made perfect sense when all the sounds and shapes we would come across adults were already around us at birth, but it had some unexpected implications for reading.

Modern forms of writing have come about through the overlaying of myriads of decisions across the centuries, but the cortex of all the decision-makers would already have undergone their preliminary tuning. Consequently, their choices appear to have favoured symbol shapes (e.g. letters) with the visual properties of more everyday sights. Symbols were chosen that could most easily be told apart by a visual system trained on the natural world. The symbols used in all languages can be represented by a limited number of strokes (usually three or less) which can be arranged in different ways. The frequency of these different arrangements corresponds to the frequency with which they occur in natural scenes (e.g. animal and human figures seen against natural landscapes).[515] In other words, our symbols were chosen by a brain that expected a world without symbols.

Reading involves connecting different types of information

Reading is, of course, much more than just processing visual information. When written language contains phonograms, reading requires visual symbols to be turned into speech before their meaning can be understood. In a simple "step-wise" fashion, we might think of reading as a two-stage process involving three types of information. To read, we must be able to translate visual information about the shapes of the written language (or *orthographic* information) into sounds that comprise the words (or *phonological* information), and translate this into meaning-based (or *semantic*) information. Skilled readers must activate several systems to process these different types of information.

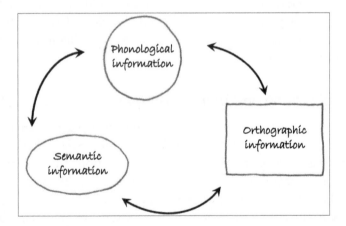

Rather than a step-wise process, however, the highly interconnected nature of the brain suggests all three types of information are being processed largely in parallel. Skilled recognition of a word happens through three streams of information coming together in a way that allows them to inform each other.[516]

Brain regions involved with the processing of these three types of information have been identified in the left hemisphere (but such examples of *lateralisation* are not evidence for left- and right-brained thinking – see box on p. 144). The function of these regions can be broadly described using the shapes above to indicate which type of information they specialise in. Some of these regions process more than one type of information (as denoted below by two shapes overlaid on each other):

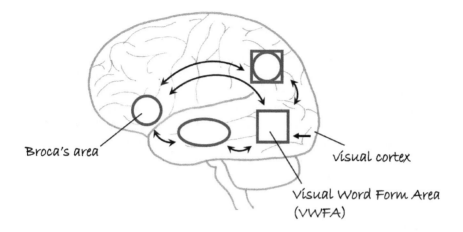

Visual information about a word first arrives into the reading network from the visual cortex. The visual word form area (VWFA) is heavily involved in recognising the orthography of the word's symbols,[517] but reading also involves the rest of the network working in parallel, drawing on semantic information (including contexts) to transform these symbols into speech sounds.[518–520] As one might expect, these processes include Broca's area – an important speech region we came across in Chapter 6 – which helps convert the phonological make-up of the word into full speech.

Learning to read and how the brain gets "re-tuned"

When we first encounter printed text as young children, we process it as we might other types of visual pattern, and we often try to recognise whole words by their overall form, engaging left and right hemispheres in the process. However, a critical step towards reading is grasping the alphabet principle, i.e. that letters, or group of letters such as "ch", represent speech sounds. Once children possess this principle and have mastered a mapping between letters and sounds, they have a self-teaching mechanism for decoding unfamiliar words into speech, and for firming up on their translation of more familiar ones.[521–523] As they practise reading, we see visual regions in the right hemisphere becoming less active and greater activation of regions involved with phonological and orthographic processing in the left hemisphere.[524] In other words, learning to read involves a slow shift from the right to the left hemisphere as our reading improves.

When learning to read begins, the brain has already undergone quite a bit of tuning during its sensitive periods. The phrase "sensitive period" refers

Left-brained/right-brained?

Language is perhaps the best known example of "laterality", when a mental ability draws unevenly on the two sides of the brain. In the case of language, the left hemisphere regions are generally more strongly involved than the right. However, even with this famous example, there are several regions in the right hemisphere that are also implicated in language, and especially when the language tasks are demanding.[525] In particular, there are regions in the right hemisphere that are strongly involved with reading comprehension[526] and the creative use of language.[527] Also, there are notable individual differences in how language is lateralised. For example, Broca's area is found in the right hemisphere in about 5% of right-handed males and, in a higher number of females, its function is distributed in both the left and right frontal cortices. Amongst left-handed people, 40% have the functions of Broca's areas distributed in both hemispheres or on the right.[528]

Misinterpretation of brain data showing lateralisation has helped produce the myth of so-called "left and right-brained thinking".[529] In fact, the largest interconnection in the brain is the corpus callosum, which acts as an information super-highway ensuring both hemispheres communicate in a sophisticated parallel fashion during even the simplest everyday tasks. Adults' phonological skills (critical for speech and reading) are predicted by levels of connectivity in the corpus callosum,[530] which would not be the case if language was an exclusively left hemisphere activity. It is difficult to find any scientific basis for the notion of left- and right-brained thinking, and categorising people as left- or right-brain thinkers takes the confusion one step further.

to a period when learning is easier, but change can still occur outside of such periods. The plasticity of the cortex may be greatest when we are young, but the existence of sensitive periods in infancy does not mean that the functional architecture of our brains is fixed by around three years old (see box opposite). The sensitive periods we know most about occur in infancy. These involve very primary functions developing in response to encounters with normal or "to-be-expected" experiences – such as seeing near and far objects, and the everyday sounds of language.

Learning to read brings about some particularly interesting changes in the region that becomes known as the VWFA but, although it's called the "visual word form area", this is not an innate reading module that we're born with. At the time when learning to read begins, this is just the brain region most suitably tuned for perceiving shapes like letters. This tuning,

The myth of three

The existence of sensitive periods in infancy has helped proliferate the so-called "myth of three", i.e. the idea that the direction of a child's development is fixed after three years old. Amongst other things, this myth has helped promote ideas about "hot-housing" normal children with highly enriched material environments and resources, in the belief this will bring about returns that are disproportionate with any later experiences. (In contrast, the evidence shows adult–child interactions and staff training are the key quality indicators of pre-school environments that influence later learning and development.)[531]

Some of the evidence used to support this myth has been drawn from studying rats in an enriched environment, and how this effected their learning and their synapses.[532,533] This is despite the researchers themselves pointing out that their enriched environment was not very enriched. It was an incomplete attempt to mimic a wild environment and was enriched "only in comparison to the humdrum life of the typical laboratory animal".[533]

It is true that earlier is often better for educational interventions, although the decision when best to implement an educational programme also requires consideration of the programme's aims and content, and who will receive it.[534] Our general lifelong ability to learn reflects the continuing malleability of our brains throughout our lives. Learning to read is a dramatic example of a re-tuning after infancy that shows how plastic the brain remains beyond the early years. Evidence is now accruing for the existence of sensitive periods during adolescence.[535,536]

however, has happened while sensitive brain regions have been processing visual scenes mostly devoid of print. The VWFA activates for reading because our earliest infant history has, as it happens, resulted in it being best for the job. It is already useful for discerning small features using sharp central (or *fovial*) vision[537] and for detecting simple geometrical shapes of the type seen in letters.[538] It does not activate because it evolved for reading. Since reading requires turning these letter shapes into representations of speech, it is no coincidence that the region that becomes the VWFA also has fast connections to other parts of the brain involved in spoken language.[539,540] Again, however, rather than evolving, these connections may arise from this region's involvement in "reading" faces as infants, and from using that information to understand speech sounds.[517] It is learning to read that causes this part of the brain to specialise in the automatic and rapid recognition of letter strings, which is the first step for mapping these strings to speech sounds.[541]

As a child or adult first learns to read, activation in the region that will become the VWFA is mild but it gradually strengthens as this brain region becomes fully sensitive to the printed word, which occurs at around 10 years old. However, the tendency for the cortex to "tune in" means other types of input have already influenced this area and are "competing" for its sensitivity. Consequently, learning to read has implications for how the brain processes these other inputs. This was shown in a study of what happens in the brain when illiterate adults are learning to read. The brain region usually referred to as the VWFA in literate adults increased its activation in response to print while decreasing its response to input such as faces.[542] At the same time, a region on the opposite (right) hemisphere substantially increased its sensitivity to faces – presumably to help compensate for losses on the other side. Learning to read, then, does not just reorganise our brain for reading, but for the processing of faces too.[543]

How this reorganisation affects behaviours other than reading is the subject of ongoing research, but some evidence suggests that becoming an expert reader results in less automatic holistic processing of the whole face, and a more analytic approach to recognising faces based on their features.[544] Also, learning to read interferes with "mirror invariance" – the tendency of primates to recognise images as identical even when they are mirror images of each other. For most problems in the natural world, distinguishing between objects that are mirror images is not that helpful. If two asymmetric lions were chasing you, would it help you to distinguish between them? On the other hand, it can be quite important for a reader to distinguish between mirror letters, such as "b" and "d", and not get "bog" and "dog" mixed up. Becoming literate tends to reduce mirror invariance,[545–547] enhancing our ability to tell the difference between mirror images.[548]

Dyslexia, the cultural-genetic lag and "normality"

When the brain function of those with reading difficulty is compared with more typical readers, researchers tend to report under-activation of the systems more towards the rear (posterior) regions of the brain.[520] In the frontal regions, some studies also report under-activation[549] but more often over-activation,[520,550] which may be due to efforts to compensate.

Given that the brain is plastic, and the result of our genes interacting with our environment, such studies should not be taken as evidence that reading difficulties (including behaviours diagnosed under the label "dyslexia") are biologically determined and fixed. This is clearly demonstrated by the extent to which reading difficulties can be improved by effective educational interventions. Differences in how those diagnosed with dyslexia process sensory information in their brains may be simply due to reduced reading experience as a result of their reading difficulties.[551]

Several studies have explored interventions in terms of their effect on reading difficulty and on brain function. The types of educational strategies helpful for those with a reading difficulty resemble those suitable for readers without such a diagnosis. Interventions include focusing on phonological training,[552-554] awareness of how word parts contribute to word meaning (morphology)[555] or a combination of multiple approaches.[556] Generally, children show an improvement in reading alongside positive changes in brain activity. Differences between studies may reflect how well the approaches match the needs of individual readers in different ways, and future research may involve tailoring approaches to students' particular reading issues. The interventions generally improve the performance of "normal" readers in these studies as well, echoing the results of brain imaging studies of interventions for dyscalculia.[488] This adds to growing scepticism about the scientific value of labels such as "dyslexia" and "dyscalculia".[557]

It is interesting to consider this issue of labelling individual difference from an evolutionary perspective. Over just the last few thousand years, we have culturally inherited a massively changed environment and ever-more powerful means to transform it further. However, our genetic basis is clearly less transformed and our interaction with this new world involves acquired cultural tools. These tools, such as numeracy and literacy, use our "old" biology in new ways. In the past, before this recycling, some patterns of genetic variation across our species may have been unproblematic. More speculatively, they may even have been occasionally helpful – until, that is, a generation was required to read and perform processes such as long division.[558] It may seem less surprising, then, that quite a few of us have difficulty with these relatively recent changes in our cultural environment and the novel demands they place on us. These new demands include associating sounds and number sense with written symbols in the early years of our development. As a species, it seems unlikely we should be perfectly adapted for these and the other mental procedures and neural processes involved with numeracy and literacy. In other words, the demands of our progressive culture have advanced beyond our evolved genetic abilities to meet them.

We have already seen that such a cultural-genetic lag may exist for spoken language ability. Some evidence for this arises from the prevalence of specific language impairment (SLI), which may reflect a failure of natural selection in our prehistory to produce the best genes for speech (p. 114). This was explained in terms of there not being a limited set of SLI genes as such. Rather, speech ability may arise from a complex combination and interaction of many genes with each other, and with the environment, with such that an individual gene can be implicated in high and low-ability outcomes. The same argument holds for other cognitive functions, including those that underlie numeracy and literacy. These skills, until very recently, have involved far too small a proportion of the human population to be implicated in any genetic evolution of our species. This makes it much more likely that a lag has opened up between our genes and our culture, with the tendency of culture to "ratchet up" demand.

On this basis, it could be said that terms such as "disorder" and "abnormal" are being applied to genetic variation that has developed over deep time and been unproblematic until we invented these new forms of communication. Instead of explanations using such terms, it might be more appropriate to say our culturally invented tools are flawed relative to those that have evolved, in the sense that they are an imperfect fit to normal genetic variation.

Numeracy and literacy: together forever

Writing expresses a symbolic system of communication suitable for thinking about the world and expressing our thoughts. While approximate arithmetic still exploits our primitive abilities with quantity and recruits left/right parietal regions, we saw in Chapter 7 that formal maths recruits left hemisphere language networks more intimately involved with language.[559] It is controversial whether spoken language is totally necessary for maths, but studies of bilinguals emphasise how language influences the way maths is coded in the brain. These studies suggest bilingual children acquire memory networks for arithmetic facts in both their languages. This would explain, for example, why practice with calculating in one language may not help greatly when calculating in the other language.[560] A recent neuroimaging study[561] even suggests our spoken language may influence how we represent quantity in our brains. This close intertwining of numeracy and language in the brain appears to echo the interweaving of their prehistoric origins. Throughout our written history, being able to write down and explain reasoning with numbers and words has been central to cultural progress. This has helped ratchet up the accumulation of knowledge, not least by reducing the likelihood of progress being lost, and by providing a more stable and explicit basis for scientific reasoning.

Untethered knowledge

Although invented by bureaucrats and accountants, written language has been mastered and perfected by storytellers, poets and artists. The incredible wonder of this cultural tool is that it allows the ideas and thoughts of those we have never met to enter our own mental world. Speech allows us to communicate about things that are not in the here and now with people who are. Writing, however, further loosens our tethering to context. It greatly expands the flow of information to include those who are not present. It allows ideas to flow across space and time, such that even the words of previous generations long dead can still be heard. These inventions have helped to drive an unprecedented increase in self-awareness amongst our species, to accumulate cultural innovation and to place an increasing emphasis on the value of knowledge and understanding.

In the last few centuries, we have begun to systemise the processes by which knowledge gets transmitted across generations. In geological time, we are at the very instant when this invention – otherwise known as "education" – is arriving. So what does education do for the learning brain, and how does it relate to our biological understanding of what we are and where we came from?

9

EVOLUTION MEETS EDUCATION

RECOGNITION OF THE ROLE OF LEARNING followed swiftly on the heels of numeracy and literacy. Formal education sprung up independently in different parts of the world, but always aimed at efficiently transmitting knowledge and understanding across generations. Around 1500 BC, the Indo-Aryans settled in Northern India and the oldest Hindu scriptures known as the Vedas (meaning "to know") were written. According to the Vedas, education was aimed at the overall development of the student. Activities focused on pupils learning to recite holy text, and the disciplined execution of duties of care towards their guru and fellow students.[562] Around the same time, in ancient China, sons of nobles were being taught the "liù yì" (Six Arts). This educational programme passed on the abilities required to enact rites, perform music, pursue archery and charioteering, and excel in calligraphy and mathematics.[563] Education was also being offered by the ancient Greeks in Athens from around 500 BC, either through attendance at school or by visits from a hired tutor. The Greek curriculum consisted of a physical education that aspired to military prowess, and an aesthetic education that provided students with an appreciation of beauty and harmony. To receive these opportunities in ancient Athens you had to be free, rather than enslaved, and male. Recognising the value of education led inevitably to it becoming a prized commodity and most of its ancient forms were associated with power and exclusivity. Today, the need to provide schooling for all children in a society is only just emerging as a global objective. For example, compulsory schooling for all children in the US and UK only came about in the nineteenth century. Even now, an estimated one in six children in low- and middle-income countries do not complete primary school.[564]

What does school do for the learning brain?

School is society's organised attempt to distribute the learning it collectively values. The modern school curriculum usually includes the "gateway" skills of literacy and numeracy, but inclusion of other topics can depend on which society we're talking about. As well as providing the knowledge and understanding defined by the curriculum, there may be less obvious and unplanned benefits of school for the learning brain. Education has the potential to improve our basic underlying mental capacities. Gaining literacy can, for example, improve working memory ability.[565,566] Those who have received education are also generally better at verbal reasoning.[567-569] That said, it is difficult to disentangle apparent improvements in brain function from all the other ways in which school can affect us. For example, schools encourage certain attitudes. These include valuing learning and achievement, especially as measured by formal tests. This means that higher performance in tests of mental ability may just reflect how education makes us more "test wise" rather than grant us enhanced brain function.[570] Such a difference in attitudes may also explain why, for example, even when schooled and unschooled children show they can learn a new rule equally well, it is the schooled children who apply it more often.[571] Education perhaps trains us to perform better in some formats but not in others. Those with education can remember 10 words spoken verbally more easily than those without education. No such differences, however, are observed when remembering black-and-white line drawings.[572] Education also appears to have little impact on our ability to recall everyday objects or those in particular categories,[573] and some researchers have concluded it has little impact on our everyday problem-solving.[574]

It appears that low levels of education, while usually a source of great disadvantage, do not necessarily indicate some type of mental deprivation or even a general lack of learning.[570] It may be more accurate to think of more- and less-educated people as having developed different *ways* of learning. This was demonstrated in a recent study that compared the working memory of members of existing hunter-gatherer communities, around half of which had attended school at some point in their lives. People with and without schooling showed similar abilities in recalling a list of words that were read out to them, but they differed in the strategies they used to do this. Those with education recalled words in the same order as they were presented, while those without education recalled words in categories that were meaningful to them.[575]

None of this detracts, of course, from the immense cultural significance of education as a tool for personal and societal improvement. Education is found to be the most crucial resource for career success[576,577] and plays a key role in reducing the risk of poverty.[578,579] Education is also associated with a wide range of health benefits linked to improved knowledge and lifestyle. Education can not only lead to greater awareness that smoking is bad for you, but also to a greater tendency to act on this knowledge.[580] Education also offers some protection to our mental abilities in old age,[581] helping us to apply and extend the benefits of health knowledge in later life. And, whether it's more about health, wealth or just the pleasure of learning, more education also predicts greater happiness.[582]

The emergence of pedagogy

Given the importance of education, it would be valuable to understand how to do it well. The theory and practice of education is sometimes referred to as pedagogy. One its first practitioners (or pedagogues) was Quintilian in the first century AD. Quintilian wrote "The Orator's Education". This was a series setting out his ideas for training young men in the skills of public speaking – essential for Roman politicians and lawyers. Quintilian was not a fan of one-to-one home tuition and promoted classroom education alongside other students as the superior method. He believed students needed persistence, practice and a skilled teacher to bring their talents to fruition.[583] He dismissed suggestions that only a few gifted individuals could benefit from education. He didn't think knowledge was innate but that it had to be acquired, and students possessed natural instincts to reason and to learn that could be harnessed for this purpose. He believed the power of memory was fundamental to education and, although this was innate, it could be improved by practice. He suggested teachers should be strict but friendly, use praise and admonishment to minimise the need for punishments, always respond to questions and make sure non-volunteers amongst the class were asked questions too. He even promoted the use of what might be called scaffolding – providing guides that supported students when learning (e.g. tracing when learning to write). These ideas are strikingly close to the type of advice provided to student teachers today. Today's teachers, like Quintilian, largely develop their theories about learning by observing and reflecting on what they see happening in their own classrooms.

Science begins to tackle learning

The accelerating progress of science in the nineteenth century soon led to a more systematic study of how we develop and learn. Evolution was an important influence on many of the early pioneers. Darwin himself, in his letter to the American Social Science Association, suggested various research studies that "would probably give a foundation for some improvement" in current educational approaches.[584] Darwin listed diverse ideas for possible studies. These included investigating the musicality of children's first utterances and the influence of a child's early interests on their later development. He also proposed exploring the effects of education on children from different racial backgrounds. Darwin believed education, or the lack of it, was the apparent cause of racial differences in the mental skills valued by his society. This contrasted with the idea, popular in his time, that these differences were somehow determined and fixed.

In laying the foundations for the scientific study of mental ability, many scientists drew on Darwin's theory as an inspiration. To begin with, this was chiefly through imagining that learning and development in some way echoed evolution. A few years after Darwin wrote his letter about education, Haeckel proposed a very literal version of this idea as "ontogeny (individual development) recapitulates phylogeny (the development of the species)".[585] Haeckel created drawings of human embryos alongside those of fishes, as representatives of our ancient ancestors. These drawings emphasised – some say slightly exaggerated – the similarities between the species. They seemed to do a good job of communicating Haeckel's basic idea, i.e. that we go through stages resembling those by which our remote ancestors evolved. Although never promoted by Darwin, this became a popular notion in the nineteenth century. James Sully, psychologist and friend of Darwin, introduced an early text book on child development by claiming "the successive stages of the mental life of the individual roughly answer to the periods of this extensive process of organisation – vegetal, animal, human, civilised life".[586] The recapitulation idea continued on, influencing the American psychologist and educator G. Stanley Hall as he lay the foundations for a science of adolescence.[587] At the beginning of the twentieth century, Hall saw parallels between late child development and the first stages of human civilisation – as they were thought about at the time. He likened children to "savages" and teenagers to nomadic wanderers.[588]

Recapitulation theory does have a common sense and attractive feel to it. After all, each of us begins as a single cell, we learn to roll and slide before walking, and then we learn to speak . . . isn't that the story of how we evolved from bacteria to *Homo* . . . sort of? However, the idea that our individual development somehow retells our evolution is as seductive as it is misleading. Modern science accepts some apparent similarity between embryos of different species, but without explaining this in ways resembling anything like Haeckel's theory. Instead, studies show many differences arise between species during the early and then late periods of embryo development (a so-called "hour-glass model of divergence"). A lack of basic body plan allows embryos to look similar, but beneath these appearances a lot of important differences are emerging.[589]

Evolution – as an analogy – was soon to inspire thoughts about children's learning processes more directly and more helpfully. In 1912, a 16-year-old biologist called Jean Piaget was publishing in the field of mollusc development, and reflecting on how the great diversity of lifeforms he was studying might have come about. Piaget considered how one type of mollusc, given the right conditions, evolved into another. He saw the process as beginning with a disturbance or change in the outside world that resulted in an imbalance between the molluscs and their environment. The process was completed when the molluscs changed to fit their environment and balance was restored. Although he began by studying the development of molluscs, Jean Piaget was to later found the field of "cognitive development" – the study of how our mental abilities develop over our lifespan. Piaget was drawn to studying children's learning as a means to understand how human thought had evolved,[590,591] but went on to become one of the most influential theorists in education. Piaget believed evolutionary processes and learning processes were linked through a tendency for an organism to regain balance with the outside world. Often, he theorised, incoming information fits with our internal model of the outside world and so this model can *assimilate* it. According to Piaget, this is our state of "equilibration". Sometimes, however, information from the outside world cannot be made to fit with our internal mental ideas (i.e. assimilation is not possible). Then, we must change our internal mental world so we can *accommodate* the new information. As in a biological system, an individual's learning and development involves his/her internal system adjusting to regain balance with the outside world. Piaget's ideas have had considerable impact on how we learn today, not least through drawing attention to the differences that may exist between individual learners.

Piaget may have been inspired by analogy between biological evolution and mental development, but he carefully avoided the idea that children recapitulated their evolution. Unfortunately, however, this and many other myths about evolution soon became established in some schools and colleges. It's important to debunk the myths before we look at how evolution can authentically help us understand how we learn.

Evolutionary myth

Neuroscientists abandoned recapitulation theory long ago, but its influence has continued in social and educational thinking. In the 1960s, the Doman-Delacato theory of development proposed that efficient brain function required acquiring specific movement skills in the correct evolutionary order.[592] According to this view, if a developmental stage was skipped, perhaps when a child learns to walk before crawling, then this could damage later development – such as the ability to learn language. In this case, the prescribed treatment might be to encourage the child to rehearse crawling movements – resembling those of our distant ancestors. This was supposed to "repattern" the child's neural connections and improve their academic progress. Scientific reviews have concluded that the Doman-Delacato theory is unsupported, contradicted and without merit,[593–596] and practical approaches based upon such ideas have been revealed as ineffective.[597] Despite this, even today, the influence of these ideas can be seen in educational kinesiology (or Edu-K, also often sold under the brand name of Brain Gym).[598] Many of the exercises in this programme attempt to repattern the brain based on the Doman-Delacato theory.[599] However, despite the lack of convincing evidence for its effectiveness[600] and flaws in its theoretical basis, the programme enjoys surprising popularity amongst teachers. Across the world, most teachers believe short bouts of coordination exercises do integrate the functions of left and right hemispheres – one of several ideas promoted by Brain Gym but with little scientific basis.[601]

Another popular idea is that we have brains "left over" from evolution, and that these can take over at inopportune moments. The blossoming of neuroscience in the 1970s raised awareness of how some brain structures appear conserved from the ancient species from which we evolved. As we have seen, this is broadly true. However, in 1978, neuroscientist Paul Maclean took things further and described his "triune brain hypothesis" in the *National Society for the Study of Education* yearbook.[602] Maclean considered the brain to comprise three formations (three "brains") that reflected our evolutionary past: the reptilian brain (including the brain stem), the paleomammalian brain (limbic system) and the neomammalian brain (including the cerebral hemispheres). Application of this theory usually involves trying to detect and influence which brain is dominating.[603] The first two parts of the brain are considered to have evolved first and are, therefore, more primitive and need to be suppressed, so giving our cerebral brain a better chance to blossom. Maclean's proposal involves a type of "directional evolution" approach, labelling brain parts in ways that appeal to human and cultural notions of progress. We have seen that direction in evolution tends to be the exception rather than the rule and, when it does occur, there is no reason to suspect it will follow something we might call progress. The general increase in our technology might be called "progress", but this has occurred alongside cultural, rather than biological change. Indeed, we saw in Chapter 3 that all vertebrates (including reptiles) demonstrate a brain structure with the three divisions of forebrain, midbrain and hindbrain. Evolution appears to have proceeded by modifying these three parts rather than by adding one on top of the other.[604] Despite these flaws, Maclean's theory spread through the many "brain-based" learning programmes of the 1980s, even cropping up more recently in theories of moral education.[605] The proliferation of myths about the brain has partly been explained by the satisfying effect of including neuroscience in an explanation (see box overleaf).

Perhaps the most alarmingly popular myth about evolution, however, is that evolution is, itself, a myth. It can be said that evolution is now as firmly established in science as the roundness of the Earth, but its existence continues to spur heated exchanges around scientific evidence and our sense of who we are as a species. Many of these exchanges echo the public disputes between scientific argument and religious belief that were witnessed in Darwin's time. Based on a survey of 24 countries, only 41% of the global adult human population currently accept evolution, with 28% professing a strict creationist religious belief about the origin of our universe and of humans.[606] Evolution is better accepted amongst more prosperous countries who invest more in education, but also where religiosity is lower. This may explain why, in the United States, only one in three adults thinks evolution is true.[606] This US trend extends to its educators, with 29% of trainers of teachers in New England considering evolution and creationism should be given equal curriculum time. In the New England study, difficulties in accepting evolution were associated with a lack of scientific understanding. Around 45% of the trainers did not know that humans are apes,[607] suggesting that education is a likely factor in people accepting evolution. Indeed, the international data identifies two significant factors, other than religiosity, that influence whether an individual will accept Darwin's theory: awareness of science and knowledge of evolution.[608] While we've been discussing how evolutionary theory might benefit education, the spread of evolutionary theory appears to benefit from education.

The allure of the brain-based explanation

Part of the reason why there are so many myths about the brain may be due to the satisfying effect of even irrelevant neuroscience in an explanation. Researchers demonstrated this effect by asking members of the public and neuroscience experts to judge their satisfaction with good and bad explanations for a range of psychological phenomena.[609] Both the experts and the public were able, on average, to rate good explanations positively and bad explanations negatively. The experts were not fooled when irrelevant neuroscience was added to both sets of explanations:

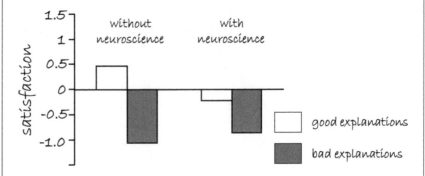

In contrast, the irrelevant neuroscience caused members of the public to generally give positive ratings to the bad explanations:

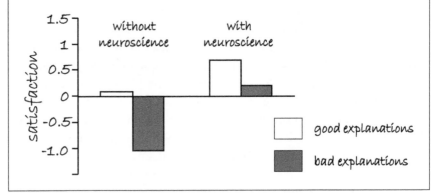

The dangers of "just so" stories?

A more recent approach to linking evolution and education has chosen a more experimental and research-based approach but − spoiler alert − this also has difficulties fitting our current understanding of how we evolved. According to the "Santa Barbara School"[191] of Evolutionary Psychology

(EP), the brain has a set of modules that do distinct things in terms of our mental processing. Some modules support specialist abilities which evolved to enhance survival or reproductive success during the Stone Age (i.e. around 2–3 million years ago). EP considers we adapted in the face of Stone Age challenges to evolve natural tendencies in specific domains. These include psychology (to understand issues such as kinship), biology (to identify plants and animals when hunting and gathering) and physics (to navigate and construct tools). EP researchers then seek out unexpected modern behaviours that still reflect these modules at work.

This has prompted some interesting experiments. For example, EP researchers suggest we may have a "cheater-detector" module sensitive to the breaking of social contracts. This module would be useful in a world dependent on social cohesion. To support this idea, EP researchers asked people to seek a relationship between information found on either side of cards. People found it easier to find the drinking rule "If a person is drinking beer, then that person must be over 19 years of age" than the rule "If a card has an 'R' on one side, then it has a '2' on the other side".[610] This might appear to suggest the social context activates additional brain power. Another group of EP researchers have argued that there are evolved sex differences in the "design features" of the jealous mind, to protect our opportunities to breed.[611] In a survey, they confirmed that when presented with different infidelity dilemmas, more men than women reported the thought of a partner's sexual infidelity (sleeping with another) to be more distressing than the thought of a partner's emotional infidelity (loving another). The idea is that this is an ancient bias that serves the male challenge of ensuring they are the father, and the female challenge of ensuring the father's investment.

This all sounds fascinating stuff but there are a variety of other, non-evolutionary and more mundane explanations for these results.[612] For example, rather than provide evidence for an evolved skill at cheater detection, we may simply learn different ways to solve abstract problems compared with those involving permission and obligation,[612] or we may interpret language differently according to the context.[613] In terms of gender differences in attitudes to infidelity, it has been pointed out that EP tends to exaggerate what we know about sex differences[614] and that the measures used by the researchers may have influenced some results.[615] Indeed, many other studies have also suggested little gender difference between responses to actual[616,617] and hypothetical infidelities.[617–619] Also, there are gender differences in how different types of infidelity predict being abandoned, so men and women may be justified in having different attitudes to these behaviours in their partners.[620] In sum, it is all too easy to create and to accept evolutionary "just so" stories, especially when we can substitute stories until one fits, without really considering entirely different kinds of explanation.[612,621] Criticism of EP has been harsh, attacking it as "the emperor's new paradigm",[612] "empirically unsupported and conceptually incoherent"[622] or just dismissing it as "potentially idle speculation".[623]

A more biological flaw with EP concerns the plastic nature of the cortex, which we've encountered many times in our history of the learning brain. This plasticity makes it unlikely we possess inherited modules for very specific types of knowledge like biology and physics. Modern behaviours that might appear innate are more likely to have come about through social and cultural influences during an individual's development. And, if one started from an evolutionary perspective, why should researchers focus on changes that occurred in the last 2–3 million years – when the epic story of our evolution lasted about a thousand times longer?

Despite these criticisms around EP itself, some think EP can inform education about why, for example, children find reading more difficult than speaking.[624,625] This, it is argued, is due to a gap between accumulating cultural knowledge and the forms of folk knowledge and abilities that emerge from children's Stone Age biases. However, although a gap between the demands of our culture and our genetic background may well exist, there is no need for this to be explained in terms of any Stone Age bias. This EP approach to education has been criticised for lacking power and falsifiability,[626] and for its lack of biological evidence.[627] To avoid the dangers of creating "just so" stories that fit modern behaviour, it seems better to start with our evolutionary history over deep time and *then* ask how this sheds light on how we learn today.

Educational learning from a deep-time perspective

Although there are many gaps, we have been able to piece together a prehistory of learning by studying the fossil record and by comparing the biology and behaviour of existing species. This tells us that 3–4 billion years of history is responsible for the incredible potential we possess to transform ourselves and our behaviour. It also emphasises that we are part of the ancient web of life rather than a freaky outlier. The arrival of ion channels, neuronal networks and the tripartite brain with features such as the basal ganglia all happened long ago in other creatures that predate our own species. Undoubtedly, we are unique – as individuals and as a species – but we owe our uniqueness to the foundational brain processes and structures that are part of a much bigger story we share with other creatures.

The deep history of our brain is the story of its slowly changing form and function. This history has limited and biased our learning abilities in some ways, while supporting them in others. We can expect the most noticeable limits and constraints in those highly valued areas of learning for which we did not evolve. These include numeracy and literacy, and many other types of formal learning experienced in schools, universities and the world of work.

More generally, the evolutionary history of our brain helps us realise how incredible our brains are. It helps us appreciate the importance of understanding how the brain functions when trying to understand and promote the ability to learn in schools, in the workplace or just for leisure. In humans, the systems discussed in Chapter 3 support many different types of learning process that allow this educational learning to take place. A student might achieve these processes independently or receive support in doing so from a teacher, but both learner and teacher can potentially benefit from understanding how these learning processes operate and how they have evolved. Let's look at three broad categories of process that are particularly relevant for education: processes supporting *engagement* for learning, *building* of knowledge and *consolidation*.

Engagement for learning

All learning begins with the learner attending to some source(s) of information or insight. A teacher, who represents one such source themselves, must be able to capture and maintain the learner's attention and judiciously direct it to whatever other sources of information and insight are helpful. There are ancient motivational and emotional biases that impact on our abilities to engage our attentional abilities, and these biases originally evolved to aid learning rather than disrupt it. Early on in our evolution as vertebrates, we evolved tendencies that bias our attention towards experiences that promise to be rewarding. Teachers offer a range of rewards that support engagement in the classroom, many of which are social ones (praise, gold stars, points etc.) that contribute to self-esteem and social standing. These types of social reward influence the brain's reward system in a similar way to other incentives such as receiving money,[628–630] food[631] or even playing video games.[632] When it comes to influencing our engagement, what is meant by the term "reward" can, therefore, be very broad.

Novelty also attracts our attention, again stimulating our reward system in a way that can increase engagement and promote learning.[633] Novel contexts can help engage students initially with a new topic, or help encourage them to apply and practise their freshly learnt knowledge in new scenarios. Topics that engage curiosity have also been shown to stimulate the brain in regions similar to those stimulated by reward.[634]

However, novelty and classroom rewards are not always necessary for engaging students because just sharing attention can, in itself, be rewarding. We have seen that our strong motivation to share attention is a uniquely human characteristic that may have played a key role in our ancient cultural accumulation of knowledge, as it does today. When self-initiated, this capturing of shared attention also leads to reward-related brain activations.[412] This suggests that just prompting someone else to share attention with you can be a desirable thing to do. It may also explain why asking students to communicate their ideas to each other in different ways can help engage their interest in learning, whether they do this through addressing the class or through helping one another in pairs to master skills.

One can, of course, expect a wide range of individual differences in how students engage with any experience. Some learners, across their lifespan, generally have more difficulty in focusing their attention in classrooms, which are settings that can demand low levels of physical activity. In these environments, such learners show a lack of concentration, short attention span and physical restlessness, and these symptoms can lead to a diagnosis of Attention Deficit Hyperactivity Disorder (or ADHD). Some scientists, however, consider these symptoms arise from genes whose common occurrence reflects the adaptive value of these traits in our evolutionary past (faster response to predators, better hunting performance, effective territorial defence and greater capacity for moving and settling).[406] This raises questions about the extent to which ADHD prevalence reflects the new social demands of our modern society. Wherever one stands in this debate, neuroimaging sheds light on the difficulties these individuals experience when trying to learn, with less activity observed in brain regions that anticipate reward.[635] Medication (e.g. methylphenidate) can enhance this reward response but research also suggests the types of strategy discussed above become even more important. Students diagnosed with ADHD benefit from a greater focus on the use of praise, prizes and privileges to encourage appropriate behaviours as well as reprimands, and an organised approach to peer-tutoring.[636]

In contrast to features of an educational experience that encourage an "approach" response, anxiety can produce avoidance of a topic and so prevent engagement. For example, avoidance is a well-established characteristic of maths anxiety. Maths-anxious students generate additional activity in regions of their amygdala associated with negative emotions and fearfulness.[124] Fear conditioning evolved to keep us safe from physical danger, but it can operate both consciously and unconsciously in ways that are problematic for classroom learning.

Learning then, and particularly our inclination to engage with it, shares ancient roots with emotion and involves biases that educators should not ignore. As importantly, we have evolved systems of communication that support the unconscious communication of these emotions. This means teachers and parents may not even know when they are transmitting emotions likely to undermine or promote the learning of others. In Chapter 4 (p. 77), we saw how the mirror neuron system can support the social learning of actions and skills, but it can also help transmit positive and negative attitudes and emotional responses. Observing an emotion in someone else (e.g. through their expression) activates some of the same brain regions involved with experiencing those emotions.[637-639] These unconscious workings of our brains help explain how easily negative emotions, such as anxiety about mathematics, can be transmitted from teacher to student,[640] and how positive teacher attitudes can become linked to higher student achievement.[641] This emphasises the importance of a teacher being able to present concepts and knowledge with confidence and enthusiasm.

The building of knowledge

Attending to sources of information in the outside world can open the door to learning, but the incoming information needs processing before a new concept is meaningfully represented in the brain. When we construct new and meaningful knowledge, different pieces of information from the world must be connected together with each other and with our prior knowledge. Constructing new thoughts and connecting these to old ones places great demand on our limited working memory – our ability to consciously attend to information.

This process of building new knowledge is perhaps the most modern part of everyday learning, benefiting from our capacity for conscious effortful thought and a range of modern, cultural supports. These supports are important because our working memory system is not greatly different to other species and its capacity in some respects is comparable to some other primates.[642] In our prehistory, beads and scratchings on bone helped us compensate for the limitations of our mental abilities. Now, we have cultural artefacts such as books and the internet to support us. These help us to extend our limited capacities, to point us towards what we should be attending to and enabling us to build up our knowledge independently. Of course, it still takes effort to consciously link together the pieces of information we need. Sometimes you might notice yourself, or another learner, after attending closely to some source of information, averting their gaze away from what's in front of them. This is thought to help us avoid distraction while making the effort to connect everything up.[643]

Although books and the internet are a great support for learning, perhaps the greatest source of support we can ever have at our disposal is a good teacher. Unlike material scaffolding, teachers can consider the internal world of the learner[644–646] and mould the information they present according to whatever they find there. They can identify the concepts that can build on the learner's present understanding and select the most appropriate way to express these. They can also use their understanding of what the learner already knows by explicitly encouraging them to make appropriate connections with their prior knowledge. This is particularly important for children, because the neural circuitry required for making these connections is still developing.[647,648] By presenting, clearly and concisely, just what's needed to meaningfully understand the concept, the teacher can reduce any unnecessary burden on the learner's working memory as they struggle to consciously put together new ideas in their mind. Differences in rates of learning and development mean that teachers need to continuously monitor what their students know and how they are thinking, and they need a good theory of mind to enable them to do this.[649–652]

The ability to teach can seem almost like a superpower. Teachers rewire and restructure the brains of others in ways that can be as biological and, ultimately, as life-changing as the effects of neurosurgery. Usually, however, teaching is carried out with much more precision in terms of the consequences for mental ability. While a surgeon seeks out a brain region with a general function, a teacher targets those neural networks in their students that encode a specific set of memories, then helps them change the connectivity of these networks in very particular ways. Through skilful interaction with our minds, a good teacher literally transforms us, mentally and biologically.

Consolidation of learning

All educational learning involves the learner engaging with information and using it to build new knowledge, but this is not the end of the story. Until consolidation, fresh knowledge is difficult to apply and vulnerable to loss. Somehow the knowledge must become more permanently embedded in our memory, and connected sufficiently to other ideas and different contexts so we can usefully apply it.

We have been evolving over billions of years to process information, rather than just to store and retrieve it. From the outset, the function of neurons was to transform incoming information and turn it into outgoing information. In other words, we have evolved to do something *with* information – not just to absorb it. Hardly surprising then that shallow processing – such as that involved with, for example, simply hearing a new word – leads to a poor memory for the word. To ensure consolidation of new information, it must be processed more deeply.

Carrying out a task that requires you to process the fuller meaning of new knowledge in different contexts is a double bonus. It can not only help you understand the knowledge better but will also help you remember it longer.[653] Testing is often used only to evaluate student knowledge but it's an effective way of ensuring this deeper processing occurs and for accelerating the rate at which learning becomes consolidated. Being tested on material makes it more likely to be remembered in the final test, and more so than simply rereading the material.[654] There is also evidence that testing slows the rate of forgetting in the longer term.[655] It works well for learning a diverse range of topics, over a wide range of education levels and for many different age groups.[656–660] All of this points towards the need to provide engaging opportunities for students to be challenged on their understanding, but in low-risk tasks that are free of anxiety (unlike formal assessments). Recent neuroimaging research suggests that repeatedly retrieving information causes it to become represented in the brain in different ways – essentially connecting it with different meanings and making it easier to retrieve in the future (see box below).[661]

Testing and the brain

A study of Swedish adults learning Swahili showed brain activation related to their new knowledge took on a greater range of forms after testing. This increased variation was seen in a region of the parietal lobe thought to act as a "convergence zone" where the different pieces of information that comprise a concept become bound together, supporting representation and storage of that concept in the brain:

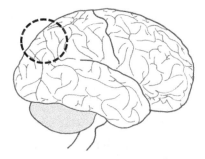

Variability here suggests testing is causing the new knowledge to be stored in a range of different ways. Just as having many different hats can make using a hat easier and more useful, so having many different versions of the new knowledge, linked to different ideas and different associations, makes it easier to find and to use later.[661] For similar reasons, consolidating knowledge and understanding is also helped by applying it in new situations, discussing it with others or expressing it in new forms. All these practices bring about new associations and meanings, helping to produce new versions of the knowledge and so make it more accessible and useful.

Interestingly, however, one primal type of information processing has received less attention from educators. In Chapter 2 we saw that the conversion of sensory information into action has been a central organising principle of the brain that predates vertebrates – but movement is rarely a priority in academic types of learning. Education may be missing a trick here. When learning words and phrases, we know that performing appropriate gestures at the same time can enhance learning, at least compared to just reading and/or listening.[662] This "enactment" effect[663–665] has been shown to work across a range of populations, including children, the elderly,[666] those with cognitive and mental impairments,[667] and Alzheimer patients.[668] However, unlike testing, the use of movement is not entirely aligned with the "sit still" ethos in many classrooms and it's easy to understand why many teachers might not be keen on the idea. But the evidence for learning through movement is accumulating. Recently, a brain imaging study has provided a little more insight into how enactment works. This has confirmed that performing a gesture when memorising a word leaves a movement "trace" in the word's representation in the brain.[669] Enactment appears to activate an additional set of brain networks partially intertwined with those involved with learning the new concept, including networks for greater attention.

Of course, some topics lend themselves to being taught through enactment more easily than others. Learning action words of a foreign language alongside experiencing the actions might sound fairly straightforward. The physics of forces can be physically experienced and literacy can be combined with drama, but how do we involve movement with, say, mathematics? However, technology is increasingly making it possible for new active learning experiences to be both created and studied more closely. In one example, dance-mats allowed children to explore numbers and quantity with their bodies. Kindergarten children were asked to compare quantities using a full-body movement on a digital dance mat, stepping to the left or right according to whether one number was larger than another. Compared with responding by ticking a box, the spatial training enhanced children's performance on a number line estimation task and on a subtest of a standardised mathematical assessment.[670] Another successful intervention in science lessons involved a mixed-reality learning environment. In a titration experiment carried out by pairs of students, learning was improved when one student added base molecules while the other added acid molecules, grabbing virtual molecules with their physical wands and then tossing them into a virtual flask.[671]

Sleep is another important part of consolidation that has been evolving at least since vertebrates began and possibly since the first central nervous system. This "price for plasticity" must be paid but many of us end up in debt, and lack of sleep is clearly linked to academic underachievement amongst children.[672,673] Adolescent learners are particularly prone to suffering a shortened sleep period after falling asleep late. This is due partly to biological reasons, with puberty disrupting circadian rhythms, but also due to increased freedom and technology use. Forced awakenings on school days add further to teenage sleep loss.[674] The result is widespread daytime teenage sleepiness and associated reductions in mental abilities such as working memory function.

In general, our evolutionary history encourages a shift in how we view learning and education to a perspective that includes our biological basis. This perspective gives strong emphasis to some concepts, such as emotion, attention and action, that are less emphasised in educational thinking – at least in respect of their significance for learning.

Evolution and a science of learning

The other important way that evolution can help education is by providing a stimulus and framework for scientifically researching, understanding and thinking about the brain in education. To meet the challenge of bridging brain science and education, a new field of research emerged at the beginning of this century. It is still young, however. So young, in fact, that researchers have still to settle on a name for it. It gets referred to as "Neuroeducation", "Educational Neuroscience" or sometimes "Brain, Mind and Education", with the "mind" emphasising how psychology is key to all these ventures.[675] This new area of research is using methods from classroom observation to brain imaging to develop a "Science of Learning" for education. Research centres combining neuroscience, psychology and education are springing up around the world, together with postgraduate and professional training for teachers.

Researchers in these centres are focusing on *how* we learn, and *how* some strategies help us learn more effectively than others. The emphasis on "how" reflects a belief that learning cannot be improved by just prescribing "what works". A student's learning is impacted by where they are learning, what they are learning and already know, their cultural background and many other factors. Few prescriptions are likely to exist now or in the future that can be guaranteed to improve learning outcomes whatever the learner and their situation. Indeed, teachers rarely try to apply a "one size fits all" approach to their students. Instead, they constantly adapt their teaching to the learner and the context, apply their own theory about their students' mental processes and so decide how best to scaffold these processes.[646] Possessing a scientific understanding of how these processes operate is important for teachers when developing their approach. It's been said that trying to teach without a scientific understanding of learning is a bit like trying to fix a washing machine without knowing how it works[676] and students, most would agree, are much more complex than washing machines. Currently, however, there are very few examples of initial teacher education that include an understanding of how the brain learns. This lack of educational focus on learning processes gives a sense of the distance that education must travel in the years ahead. It also helps explain the global prevalence right now of myths about the brain that are associated with poor classroom practice.[601]

The relating of neuroscience to learning in colleges, classrooms and the workplace is not entirely straightforward. For one thing, there are big differences in concepts and language between neuroscience and education. This gap between neuroscience and education provides an obvious challenge when "making meaning" of our neurobiology in an educational sense, i.e. identifying key messages about what the neuroscience means for everyday learning and, as importantly, what it doesn't mean. However, evolution can aid this process of sense-making by guiding attempts to understand our learning brain through comparing it to that of other species. This guidance includes clues as to the primal and foundational nature of some brain processes compared with others. For example, the time frame of evolution gives more emphasis to vertebrate emotional biases than any alleged Stone Age modular bias. In this way, evolution can also help identify the types of bias that might be targeted by future research. Evolution helps us understand how our brain was shaped and what it was shaped to do, and may provide an alternative perspective on difficulties with cultural inventions such as numeracy and literacy. Finally, the inclusion of an authentic understanding of evolution in educational thinking can provide a first defence against evolutionary "neuromyth". In all these ways, evolution may prove vital for attempts to inform educational thinking, policy and practice with insights into how the brain learns.

10

THE FUTURE OF THE LEARNING BRAIN

S O HERE WE ARE at zero hour – the present day – that precious moment snatched between past and future. In one rotation of our 24-hour clock, we have covered 3.5 billion years of evolutionary time. Would it be mad to try and peek an instant into the future . . . perhaps just one-hundredth of a second on our evolutionary clock . . . about 400 years of real time . . . ?

Much of our future will depend on the decisions made by our species and, from a scientific point of view, predicting the big decisions of just one individual is immensely difficult. In theory, with perfect knowledge, we could make such a prediction based on a person's genes, past experiences and the situation they find themselves in. Of course, we simply don't know enough to make such predictions with accuracy and, even if we did, we'd probably never have a computer powerful enough to calculate someone's destiny from birth. But then think about predicting what a global population will do over the next 400 years – considering all the possible interactions between those individuals! Clearly, science has no crystal ball for predicting the future of our species.

However, science can draw attention to some of the key drivers that might influence our future over the next few centuries, and help us identify some of the options. One evolutionary event on the rise right now is *extinction*. Our own future is intimately bound up with those of other species, and we have clear evidence these are disappearing at an unusual and alarming rate. This disappearance is due largely to the expansion of our own population. Populations cannot expand forever; resources are limited and change is inevitable. Our future decisions and actions will greatly influence whether most forms of life, including our own, will avoid the very real and imminent threat of extinction.

But what about *evolution* rather than extinction – is it possible our genetic background might evolve in the future and positively influence our decisions? Across deep time, we have often seen evolutionary change occurring alongside environmental change, and the human environment has been dramatically transformed in recent years by tools such as the internet. This makes it sound plausible that our increasingly intense culture might itself be a new and powerful driver for genetic change, one that could help us evolve to make decisions that are better for our future.

On the other hand, perhaps technology may affect us in ways that circumvent the usual evolutionary processes. After all, technology can already provide *enhancement* of our human abilities without involving natural selection. Could such enhancement impact on the course of our evolutionary history – by supplementing our biology, improving how we live, think and operate, and so helping us to avoid extinction? And then, of course, there is *education*. What role might our most powerful political tool for learning have in all this?

Amongst the infinite range of futures we might face, let's take a glimpse at just four imagined scenarios – selected to explore some of the factors bound up with the future of the learning brain: extinction, evolution, enhancement and education.

Scenario 1: extinction

In 400 years' time, the average temperature of the planet is several degrees higher. Most vertebrate species are already extinct and the severe loss of biodiversity has taken whole eco-systems with it. Crop pollination and water purification are now all but impossible. In a world of shrinking resources, relationships between nations become characterised by distrust and conflict. Modern warfare greatly exacerbates global pollution, accelerating the loss of diversity and sealing the fate of our own species. If H. sapiens still exists at this point, it will not survive to witness the other side of an irreversible mass extinction.

Many scientists had become optimistic that a pause in the rate of global warming was occurring in the first 15 years of the present century. Sadly, however, recent data has dashed those hopes. It appears the apparent pause was really down to underestimating ocean temperatures over the last two decades. With this correction, the temperature of our planet is rising by around 0.07 to 0.12 degrees per decade, with an increasing rate of warming in recent years:[677]

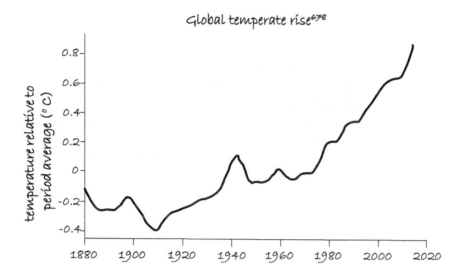

Global temperate rise[678]

Along with the temperatures, many species are also on the move in ways never seen before. Britain's south coast is seeing gilt-head bream coming from the open sea into its estuaries, young wasp spiders are appearing in Northern Europe and small red-eyed damselflies are appearing in greater numbers throughout the south of England. Canadian polar bears, who usually depend on a frozen sea, are spending longer on land. Quiver trees in South Africa are shifting away from the Equator and umbrella trees are moving northwards in the US. Temperatures are climbing and the world is changing.

A few species may benefit and even see their populations expand as part of these changes, but others will increasingly become part of the largest mass extinction seen for 65 million years. The rate at which species have been disappearing over the last few hundred years is unprecedented in human history. Even against the geological timescale of Earth's history, the accelerating rate of extinctions is highly unusual. If it continues even for a few more human lifetimes, it will become effectively permanent. Based on the five previous events that might be compared with the present sixth extinction, life will take hundreds of thousands to millions of years to recover its diversity.[679]

And the point of no return, if not already passed, may not even take a few lifetimes to reach. Withholding the destructive capacity of our species depends on a fragile political stability. In 1947, two years after the destruction of Hiroshima and Nagasaki, the scientists who created the nuclear bomb drew up the Doomsday Clock. This is a symbol which represents the likelihood of global catastrophe. Every year, the board of scientists meet to decide whether its hands should be moved closer to or further from midnight – the point at which catastrophe is unavoidable. At the time of writing it is set to 2½ minutes to midnight, the closest we have been to ultimate disaster since 1953.[680] The board cites the rise of nationalism, the refusal of the US administration to accept the scientific consensus over climate change, the US President's comments over nuclear weapons and the threat of a renewed Russia–US arms race.

If extinction is to be avoided, our species must learn to change its behaviour fast enough to escape these advancing threats. But how might this come about? Could we, for example, be evolving to learn more readily? It doesn't sound too implausible that the culture that has so empowered our learning brain might also be evolving it.

Scenario 2: evolution

In 400 years' time, alongside mounting environmental and political challenges, our learning brain has evolved to fit a cultural world of 24/7 digital technology and almost unlimited access to information. This has driven up our IQ and provided us with the additional mental resources required to maintain the planet's biodiversity and secure our own survival.

While evolution generally lacks an overall direction, cultural behaviour has driven us towards increased sophistication and greater efficiency, empowering us to make an increasingly greater impact on the world around us and how we experience it. Whether or not we wish to call this "progress", it reflects a certain direction of travel and so raises an interesting possibility. If this direction has been favouring some mental process over others, perhaps this new cultural world has been creating new pressures for our learning brain to evolve. It's certainly not very smart to be destroying our habitat – but will we be more genetically predisposed to smartness in the future?

Some evidence does suggest we have been getting cleverer over the last century. Soon after the intelligence quotient (or IQ) was developed early in the twentieth century, it was being used to appoint employees, accept military personnel and award university places. This is because IQ correlates with a range of measures of academic and professional success, as well as improved health and life expectancy. Once average IQ scores within populations began to be measured, they could be compared year by year. By the middle of the century, it was clear scores were rising. At first, scientists saw this as a statistical anomaly, shrugging off the idea that we were getting smarter.[681,682] However, systematic approaches in the 1980s confirmed what has since become known as the "Flynn effect": IQ scores were generally increasing over generations, with one analysis showing an average increase of about three IQ points per decade.[683]

It is tempting to think our brain has been genetically adapting to keep pace with our ever-more demanding modern culture. Studies of animals hint that genetic changes in mental ability can occur rapidly. For example, after foxes were selected for tameness over a mere 40-year period, scientists observed an inherited shrinking of their skulls.[684] Since there is a correlation between brain size and IQ, such changes could reasonably have implications for mental ability. We certainly have evidence of culture impacting on the genetics of diet and disease. Dairy farming, for instance, coincided with the arrival of lactose tolerance,[685] and some populations have become more resistant to malaria in places where mosquitoes proliferate[686,687] – such as near tyre factories, where they infest the rainwater collecting inside the tyres.[688] We know culture can impact on brain evolution via diet and disease (see box below), but could there be a more direct route?

Sexual selection might, in theory, help skew the genetic profile of a population towards smartness. We know modern-day humans do show a preference for an intelligent mate when choosing a partner and this preference could, hypothetically, have promoted increases in intelligence over generations.[689] However, in industrialised society, this appreciation of greater intelligence is probably offset by less interest generally in reproducing. We see only a negative association between IQ and reproduction, and this predicts a drop in IQ points of about 0.8 points per decade. For

---

Culture's impact on evolution over recent millennia

Scientists have been checking whether genetic changes related to diet and disease might also have influenced brain evolution. This would be another, albeit indirect way in which culture may have impacted on the genetic basis of our mental abilities. In 2005, there was excitement when scientists found changes in two types of allele that may have occurred in the last few thousand years: microcephalin and abnormal spindle-like microcephaly-associated protein (ASPM).[690,691] Since both alleles were thought to affect brain development,[692] these recent evolutionary changes might also have influenced intelligence. Subsequent work has shown that the microcephalin allele does indeed correlate with IQ across different populations.[693,694] Populations with higher levels of microcephalin tend to have slightly higher IQ averages. Microcephalin is thought to be involved in DNA repair and can increase neurogenesis after influenza infections.[695] It may, therefore, have been selected for through its special role in anti-viral immune response, protecting the brain when a virus strikes. By reducing the spread of disease, this gene may have become indirectly responsible for raising a population's IQ.[696]

women, at least, this is irrespective of education. Women in the UK with greater intelligence have been becoming more likely to choose childlessness over the last half-century.[697]

As it turns out, we no longer consider IQ as wholly determined by genetics and the Flynn effect can be explained without the involvement of evolution. IQ can be increased by socio-economic advantage, a stimulating environment, parental attitudes, maternal age and education[279] – all of which may have helped IQ scores to creep upwards over time. Acquiring gateway skills such as reading open the door to additional intellectual stimulation, explaining how reading ability in the early teenage years predicts future increases in intelligence.[698] Some interventions have focused only on rehearsing working memory and this appears to improve IQ over just a few weeks.[699,700] This potential for experience to change our IQ suggests everyday occupations may have played a role in the Flynn effect, if these have been encouraging us to practise mentally challenging tasks. In sum, scientists now explain the Flynn effect in terms of modern life providing more people with enough nutrition, medical care and other resources to slow down our life history and find more time to educate and stimulate ourselves. We now take longer to live our lives and breed, providing more opportunity to cultivate our mental abilities and raise our IQ.[701] On that basis, if the Flynn effect does not mean we are changing genetically, it would be unreasonable to expect it to continue forever. Most recently, it has been found that IQ scores may be levelling out and, in some countries, even going into reverse.[702] In short, however mentally taxing we find the culture we have created, it is unlikely to drive great changes in the genetic evolution of our brain over the next 400 years.

So, should we really dismiss the influence of modern-day culture on our brain evolution? If we're talking about evolution through changes to our DNA, then maybe so, but *epigenetics* offers another way in which the environment can impact on our inherited abilities (see box opposite). In studies of rodents, different types of parent–infant interactions bring about a range of epigenetic changes in the brain. These are particularly in the hippocampus, which is a key area for learning.[703] For example, infant mice who become separated from their mother show impaired social behaviour, but also increased DNA methylation in genes for producing cortisol – a stress hormone.[704] The epigenetic changes and behaviours persist into the next generation. These can be adaptive. If the high-threat environment continues into the next generation, the rodents are born already biologically prepared for stressful situations. Otherwise, if the threat does not continue, they are a potential source of vulnerability, since they provide a poor fit to a more benign world. These are very early days for human epigenetic research, but

Epigenetics: a "new" new synthesis?

Recently, scientists have begun to consider whether evolution may not be all about DNA. In some important respects, organisms can also adapt to their environment by switching genes on and off rather than changing them. This is called *epigenesis*. For example, an organism's experience of the outside world can cause a methyl group (CH3) to bind to part of the DNA and make that part less functional. In this way, by switching certain genes on an off, an individual organism can achieve a biological "fit" to the environment quite rapidly during its own development. Incredibly, some of these changes appear to get passed on to the next generation. Despite the modifications being inherited, the DNA itself does not change, just its expression.

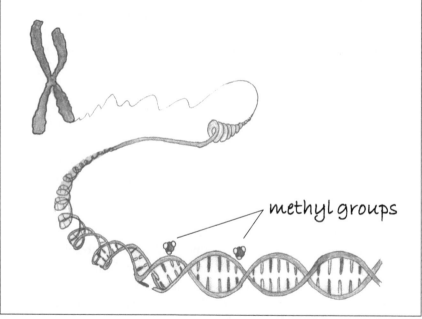

methyl groups

there is good reason to expect similar mechanisms to operate for our own species when we encounter adverse environments.[705] Cortisol secretion alters in children who suffer early adversity[125] and, when stress occurs in pregnant women, research has shown their change in cortisol levels can be passed on to their children.[706] The growing understanding of how toxic stress can be passed biologically down generations will hopefully help find ways to prevent or reduce the damage it causes.[707]

We have, however, barely begun to scratch the surface of what epigenetics means for the learning brain. At the time of writing, we have no evidence of any epigenetic enhancement of IQ that can be passed down generations. Nonetheless, for many scientists, epigenetics feels like a game-changer. It reveals much more of a two-way interaction between nature and nurture than was originally thought possible. Referring back to the days when genetics first met evolutionary theory, there are now calls for a new "new synthesis" that includes genetic and epigenetic adaptation.[708]

Scenario 3: enhancement

After another 400 years of progress in technology and science, the biological basis of human intelligence has become enhanced. Electrical and chemical stimulation is improving brain function, and communications technology has merged with our nervous system, supporting the sharing of emotional experience across global digital networks. When famine strikes one part of the world, those on the other side of the planet feel the pain and suffering too, prompting immediate relief efforts and a global sense of hope. Every individual is a single component in a worldwide network of human experience. The human species is beginning to operate as a single community. We can prioritise broad, long-term goals of universal planetary significance, assuring survival of our species and the environment on which we depend. Moreover, again aided by technology, the species is editing its own genome, eliminating defects and improving our biological fit to the new world we are creating.

One difficult area to extrapolate into the future is where technology is taking us. This is despite the popularity of this topic in science fiction. The above scenario has its roots in what is currently possible. Arguably, it takes a very optimistic stance on how existing types of technology will be improved and distributed in the future.

Brain-enhancing drugs, such as Methylphenidate and Modafinil, are currently only available on prescription but they are now being used by healthy individuals who purchase them over the internet. Surveys of students reveal usage rates of between 2% and 16%.[709] The journal *Nature* received 1,400 responses from an online poll in which one in five respondents reported having used these types of drugs chiefly to improve concentration and focus. A similar rate of use was reported amongst 1,200 German-speaking surgeons who attended a conference in 2011. It is difficult to be sure whether current usage is increasing, although it seems reasonable to assume that future stimulants will become more powerful and cheaper to produce.

Transcranial electric stimulation (TES) is another method for enhancing brain function and involves small currents being applied across the scalp. TES has a history extending back to the beginning of the nineteenth century[710] but it has recently been attracting renewed interest. This is chiefly because scientists have begun to identify the optimal size, type and location of current required to impart different cognitive effects and to understand how these effects operate.[711] In a modern study, the military potential of TES was assessed using a virtual reality training game that familiarised personnel with a Middle-Eastern threat environment before they were deployed.[712] Adult volunteers who received 2 milliamps to the scalp showed twice as much improvement in learning and performance as those receiving one-twentieth the amount of current. A few other studies of TES have recently emerged that are focused on more conventional educational aims. In one of these, three times as many adult participants achieved success in an insight problem-solving task when using TES.[713] In another adult study, a six-day course of training adults with TES produced improvement in numerical abilities that were present six months later.[714] The simplicity of the treatment for the size and duration of the effects appears remarkable, but the risks[715] and ethical implications[716] are still to be fully explored.

As well as improving our ability to reason and remember, new technologies may also help us feel more connected. Although we have seen the size of human communities increase over time, this increase does not represent a change in the intimate group size that Dunbar's limit is concerned with (see Chapter 4, p. 71). Large Facebook networks contain large numbers of fairly superficial friendships. These are the types of loose social ties that have enabled us to organise around projects on a massive scale, both constructive and destructive, but have created communities whose members may not always feel emotionally connected with each other. We saw earlier, for example, that social networking using current technology fails to increase the number of intimate friendships we can maintain. Suppose, however, that future technology could help us expand intimate communication and sharing of our feelings over much larger networks, so that we can better feel what others feel, but on a massive scale.

Both digital technology and our nervous system, including our brain, operate using electrical signals. If the brains of individuals could be connected directly to the internet, this might allow a merging of the two processing systems and a massive extension of the brain's processing capabilities. These capabilities could include neural communication between individuals who are online. This has been demonstrated in a rudimentary way by Kevin Warwick who had a microelectrode array surgically implanted into the nerve fibres of his left arm.[717] When his wife also had electrodes implanted into her left arm, the couple were able to connect their nervous systems across the web. This was the first demonstration of merging digital and human information networks and, although somewhat primitive, it demonstrates the basic principle. When Warwick generated a neural impulse by moving his finger, this could be sensed by his wife and vice-versa. Effectively, then, connecting nervous systems across the internet allows for the sharing of intimate experience more directly and widely than is currently possible, wherever the connected individuals might physically be located. One can extend this further to imagine how the neural signals from many humans could be combined and distributed, allowing a much greater sharing of experience and consciousness.

Another very plausible way in which technology may impact on our biology is through the direct editing of our genome (see box opposite). In the short term, this would allow us to remove traits from the population that are related to disease and dysfunction. In the longer term, this would allow us to effectively take control over our own evolution.

At the moment, a variety of legal obstacles prevent scientists from pursuing gene-editing as a means to change the human genome, but the rules vary from region to region. Laws in Europe are generally very limiting. In the UK, however, while genetically modified embryos cannot be implanted into women, licenses can be obtained to alter embryos in research labs and then destroy them. There is no law banning genome-editing of embryos in the US, although the government does not fund it. In 2015, Chinese scientists announced they had successfully carried out the first gene-editing of human embryos.[718] Despite destruction of what was produced, the Chinese study showed how feasible it has become to edit the genome, igniting a serious ethical debate.[719,720] Reports suggest four other Chinese groups are engaged with similar research.[721] In theory, these advances have made a eugenics approach much more practically achievable, with the very real possibility that *H. sapiens* might, in the future, direct its own evolution.

One can imagine many contrived and misguided financial and ideological motivations for producing an "improved" version of our species. Amongst enthusiasts of such tampering, there are complaints that "progress via Darwinian evolution is extremely slow and the direction unpredictable, save only that it will facilitate gene survival".[722] Although experts have insisted evolution does not follow the direction of what we commonly regard as progress or, indeed, much of any direction at all, the author of this quote argues we should use gene-editing to ensure that it does. He describes his own vision of what such progress would entail. His ideas for potential improvement begin innocuously with eradication of disease but then suggest new capabilities for our species: "We surely need to accelerate the development of better resistance to bacteria, disease, viruses, or hostile environments, or of the technologies that will be eventually necessary to

Gene-editing and evolution

Technology will soon allow modification of the human genome. Gene-editing is the focus of intense research effort because it promises new ways to treat many diseases, including HIV/AIDS, haemophilia, sickle-cell anaemia and cancer. Current aims are to modify the genetic material of cells other than sperm and egg cells involved with reproduction, resulting in changes only to the single individual. However, knowledge has now advanced far enough to allow editing the genome of unborn children in ways that could be passed on to future generations.

Scientists have learnt how to do this by studying how some bacteria have a primitive immune system in which a gene-editing mechanism protects them from viruses. This process involves an enzyme called Cas9 that, guided by a small piece of RNA, can cut two strands of the viral DNA at a specific location. Scientists have learnt to use a similar approach on other types of DNA, including the DNA found within a fertilised egg.

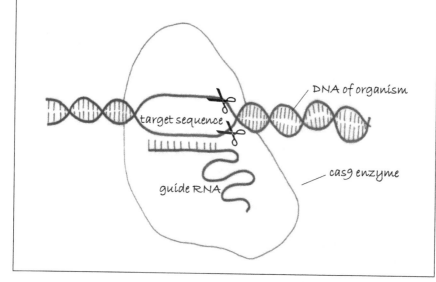

find, and travel to, habitats alternative to Earth".[722] This demonstrates, perhaps, how easy would be the slide from allowing modifications aimed at remedying disadvantage to those that produce an elite with new and special abilities. The potential of gene-editing seems perilously close to enabling the eugenics imagined by Darwin's half-cousin Galton, who wanted a science "to give to the more suitable races or strains of blood a better chance of pre-vailing speedily over the less suitable". Arguments for how science should be applied often reflect the current prevailing values of society, and Galton's approach echoed the imperial attitudes of his day. Today's argument, published in the *American Journal of Bioethics*, is couched in more neo-liberal terms, with an emphasis on individual choice:

> Once a new and beneficial technology has been demonstrated to be "safe enough" for use in or by humans, any decent society will wish to ensure that citizens are not denied the opportunity to choose for themselves whether they wish to avail themselves of these benefits.[722]

Would a population with all these technological advantages be more cohesive, and more capable of the collective action required to protect the global community and its environment? Well, possibly − and 400 years seems a reasonable time over which such technology might develop. A sceptic might point out, however, that individual access to such technology might come with a significant price tag, and we already have a global digital divide that suggests it might not be readily available to everyone. The extent to which technology might empower those able to access it needs to be balanced by the divisiveness of having large proportions of the population who could not. It seems very questionable whether such technology would be distributed well enough to help us as a species.

Scenario 4: education

The vast majority of the Earth's human population has achieved a level of political and social unity that allows it to tackle the global threats to its survival. Underpinning this sense of global community is a core of knowledge, values and understanding that is almost universally distributed. This is integrated with the learning that characterizes the individual peoples and cultures that comprise our species. In this way, we are maintaining cohesion but also assuring our diversity and creativity. A global culture has emerged capable of limiting conflict, climate change and loss of biodiversity at levels that no longer threaten a catastrophe of our own making.

Right now, the idea of something like a sense of community on a planetary scale may seem almost unattainable. However, over time, a general trend has emerged in which the size of community that humans can sustain has increased. Rather than evolution, it has been culturally based transmission and cultural development that have helped us to sustain these larger networks. This has allowed us to flourish and survive in unprecedented numbers, within strong, stable communities that tend to resist internal conflict. The size of human communities has expanded to populate village farms, cities and then nations. It is not impossible, therefore, that a fully functioning and strong global community of *H. sapiens* may one day come about – if we can innovate the methods of cultural transmission required to sustain it.

There are few organised attempts to improve the cultural transmission of knowledge, values and understanding that do not come under the heading of "education". On an individual level, education provides many benefits – and these offer knock-on effects for others within the individual's network. Better education relates to better employment outcomes and higher wages,[723] and helps us to make better decisions when we do encounter hard times.[724] Education is also one of the strongest determinants of health,[725] and children who are educated live longer and healthier lives as adults.[726,727] A health effect of education exists irrespective of a country's level of development.[728] The effects of education on health are particularly strong for young women, whose every year of additional education reduces the probability of their child dying before five years old by around 8%.[729] All these advantages for the individual also help the community. Having better-paid individuals means increased tax revenues, healthier individuals means less spending on healthcare, and reduction in inequality and poverty reduces political tension and conflict. Education can, however, have more direct benefits for the community. Education appears to make us generally more concerned with social welfare[730] and this also causes us to behave in a more environmentally friendly manner. Mixed or integrated schooling of children from politically opposed communities has a positive effect on attitudes, chiefly through children being able to experience sustained contact with each other.[731]

Education, then, really does seem vital for ensuring the well-being of human society and our planet. There may not be a panacea for the problems we are facing, but education is probably the closest thing we have to one. Also, happily, there are some signs of global progress on this front. Between 1970 and 2009, the years of schooling for women in developing countries had more than tripled, from 2.2 to 7.2 years, saving the lives of an estimated 4.2 million children.[726] However, there are still an estimated 15 million children (of which 10 million are girls) who will never go to school, and will not gain access to the "gateway" cultural tools of literacy and numeracy. The effects of such inequality are often doubly unfair, since the disadvantaged stand to reap greater benefits from education than those who are more fortunate.[732]

There is, also, a growing realisation amongst many governments that schooling is not the same as learning. Learning in school requires good-quality teaching. This is as true when children are learning the traditional curriculum as when they are learning about health, the environment and peace. For example, for education to reduce conflict, the teacher's role may be critical in enabling opportunities for children to mix and make friends of their own choosing across a political divide.[733] The evidence for global improvements in quality of education is more mixed than for school attendance. Exam results provide some indication of this quality and, on this basis, the developing world still lags badly behind. Around half or more of children completing primary schooling in many countries, including India, Bangladesh, Pakistan, Kenya and Tanzania, are unable to read even the simplest texts or perform simple arithmetic. At the current rate of progress, it will be well over 100 years before students in developing countries can produce similar results in science exams to today's students elsewhere.[734]

The likelihood of salvation through technology and science alone seems faint, and the story of the lone scientist who can save the world is likely to remain a work of fiction. Rather than the creation and retention of knowledge by a minority of experts, it seems the organised distribution of knowledge through education may be the ultimate challenge that decides our fate. Tackling big issues such as climate change, population control, conflict, mass displacement and disease all require knowledge to be dispersed amongst the wider population. Like all species, one day we will become extinct – but poor education, it seems, has the potential to hasten our departure.

The future of the learning brain

What really happens to our species, of course, will probably be a messy combination of some of the above scenarios, along with a variety of other events that could never have been foreseen. But the scenarios do serve to emphasise how much of our future will depend on learning and, if that's the case, we need to find a new sense of rigour and urgency in how we go about it. For a long time, progress in understanding and developing new methods of learning has lagged behind human accomplishment in other areas. While transport has moved from the horse to the spaceship, and medicine has moved from leeches to stem cells, changes in our approaches to learning have been modest. New scientific technologies and concepts, particularly from neuroscience, may help bring about much-needed change. Neuroimaging, for example, now allows us to study brain function during the act of learning. Mobile devices for detecting changes in electrical brain activity will soon allow neural data to be collected during learning in classrooms and lecture rooms. Science has already shed light on the effects of exercise, sleep and nutrition on the brain's readiness to learn and provided new insights into mathematics, reading and many other areas. Through collaborative ventures between education and the sciences of mind and brain, we may come to understand and greatly improve the underlying processes of teaching and learning.

Evolution can provide an important overarching framework for these new initiatives. It can help us understand ourselves and our own potential, as one small part of a much bigger picture. As individuals and as a society, by mastering and distributing the ability of our brains to learn, we may earn the chance to transform ourselves and our future.

REFERENCES

1 de Queiroz, K. Ernst Mayr and the modern concept of species. *Proc. Natl. Acad. Sci. U.S.A.* **102**, 6600–6607, doi:10.1073/pnas.0502030102 (2005).

2 Grant, P. R. & Grant, B. R. Evolution of character displacement in Darwin's finches. *Science* **313**, 224–226, doi:10.1126/science.1128374 (2006).

3 Grant, B. S., Owen, D. F. & Clarke, C. A. Parallel rise and fall of melanic peppered moths in America and Britain. *Journal of Heredity* **87**, 351–357 (1996).

4 Tutt, J. W. *British moths* (Routledge, 1896).

5 Kettlewell, H. B. D. *The evolution of melanism* (Clarendon Press, 1973).

6 Cook, L. M., Grant, B. S., Saccheri, I. J. & Mallet, J. Selective bird predation on the peppered moth: the last experiment of Michael Majerus. *Biol. Lett.* **8**, 609–612, doi:10.1098/rsbl.2011.1136 (2012).

7 Shanahan, T. *The evolution of Darwinism: Selection, adaptation, and progress in evolutionary biology* (Cambridge University Press, 2004).

8 Gould, S. J. *Life's grandeur* (Harmony, 1996), p. 137.

9 Desmond, A. & Moore, J. *Darwin's sacred cause: Race, slavery and the quest for human origins* (Penguin, 2009).

10 Ruse, M. Evolution and progress. *Trends in Ecology & Evolution* **8**, 55–59, doi:10.1016/0169-5347(93)90159-m (1993).

11 Hunt, G. The relative importance of directional change, random walks, and stasis in the evolution of fossil lineages. *Proc. Natl. Acad. Sci. U.S.A.* **104**, 18404–18408, doi:10.1073/pnas.0704088104 (2007).

12 Durand, J. F. Palaeontology and South African society today. *Tydskrif Vir Geesteswetenskappe* **53**, 331–345 (2013).

13 Jones, A. G. & Ratterman, N. L. Mate choice and sexual selection: what have we learned since Darwin? *Proc. Natl. Acad. Sci. U.S.A.* **106**, 10001–10008, doi:10.1073/pnas.0901129106 (2009).

14 Darwin, C. R. Letter to Mrs. Emily Talbot on the mental and bodily development of infants: report of the secretary of the department. *Journal of Social Science, containing the Transactions of the American Association* **15**, 5–8 (1882).

15 Darwin, C. R. Letter to J. D. Hooker, 1871. Darwin Correspondence Project, "Letter no. 7471," accessed on 29 August 2017, www.darwinproject.ac.uk/DCP-LETT-7471.

16 Dodd, M. S. *et al.* Evidence for early life in Earth's oldest hydrothermal vent precipitates. *Nature* **543**, 60–64, doi:10.1038/nature21377, www.nature.com/nature/journal/v543/n7643/abs/nature21377.html#supplementary-information (2017).

17 Schopf, J. W. & Kudryavtsev, A. B. Biogenicity of Earth's earliest fossils: a resolution of the controversy. *Gondwana Research* **22**, 761–771, doi:10.1016/j.gr.2012.07.003 (2012).

18 Hamilton, T. L., Bryant, D. A. & Macalady, J. L. The role of biology in planetary evolution: cyanobacterial primary production in low-oxygen Proterozoic oceans. *Environmental Microbiology* **18**, 325–340, doi:10.1111/1462-2920.13118 (2016).

19 Lazcano, A. & Miller, S. L. How long did it take for life to begin and evolve to cyanobacteria? *J. Mol. Evol.* **39**, 546–554, doi:10.1007/bf00160399 (1994).

20 Falkner, G. & Falkner, R. *The complex regulation of the phosphate uptake system of cyanobacteria* (Springer-Verlag, Berlin, 2011).

21 Snider, V. E. & Roehl, R. Teachers' beliefs about pedagogy and related issues. *Psychology in the Schools* **44**, 873–886 (2007).

22 Clark, K. B. Origins of learned reciprocity in solitary ciliates searching grouped 'courting' assurances at quantum efficiencies. *Biosystems* **99**, 27–41, doi:10.1016/j.biosystems.2009.08.005 (2010).

23 Eckert, R. & Brehm, P. Ionic mechanisms of excitation in Paramecium. *Annual Review of Biophysics and Bioengineering* **8**, 353–383, doi:10.1146/annurev.bb.08.060179.002033 (1979).

24 Kunita, I., Kuroda, S., Ohki, K. & Nakagaki, T. Attempts to retreat from a dead-ended long capillary by backward swimming in Paramecium. *Frontiers in Microbiology* **5**, doi:10.3389/fmicb.2014.00270 (2014).

25 Claessen, D., Rozen, D. E., Kuipers, O. P., Sogaard-Andersen, L. & van Wezel, G. P. Bacterial solutions to multicellularity: a tale of biofilms, filaments and fruiting bodies. *Nat Rev Micro* **12**, 115–124, doi:10.1038/nrmicro3178 (2014).

26 Koschwanez, J. H., Foster, K. R. & Murray, A. W. Sucrose utilization in budding yeast as a model for the origin of undifferentiated multicellularity. *PLoS. Biol.* **9**, e1001122, doi:10.1371/journal.pbio.1001122 (2011).

27 Yin, Z. *et al.* Sponge grade body fossil with cellular resolution dating 60 Myr before the Cambrian. *Proc. Natl. Acad. Sci. U.S.A.* **112**, E1453-E1460, doi:10.1073/pnas.1414577112 (2015).

28 Schweigreiter, R., Roots, B. I., Bandtlow, C. E. & Gould, R. M. Understanding myelination through studying its evolution. *International Review of Neurobiology* **73**, 219, doi:10.1016/s0074-7742(06)73007-0 (2006).

29 Liu, A. G., Matthews, J. J., Menon, L. R., McIlroy, D. & Brasier, M. D. Haootia quadriformis n. gen., n. sp., interpreted as a muscular cnidarian impression from the Late Ediacaran period (approx. 560 Ma). *Proc. R. Soc. B-Biol. Sci.* **281**, doi:10.1098/rspb.2014.1202 (2014).

30 Bale, R., Hao, M., Bhalla, A. P. S. & Patankar, N. A. Energy efficiency and allometry of movement of swimming and flying animals. *Proc. Natl. Acad. Sci. U.S.A.* **111**, 7517–7521, doi:10.1073/pnas.1310544111 (2014).

31 Albert, D. J. What's on the mind of a jellyfish? A review of behavioural observations on Aurelia sp jellyfish. *Neurosci. Biobehav. Rev.* **35**, 474–482, doi:10.1016/j.neubiorev.2010.06.001 (2011).

32 Albert, D. J. Field observations of four Aurelia labiata jellyfish behaviours: swimming down in response to low salinity pre-empted swimming up in response to touch, but animal and plant materials were captured equally. *Hydrobiologia* **736**, 61–72, doi:10.1007/s10750-014-1887-4 (2014).

33 Hebb, D. O. *The organization of behavior* (Wiley, 1947).

34 Bliss, T. V. P. & Lømo, T. Long-lasting potentiation of synaptic transmission in the dentate area of the anaesthetized rabbit following stimulation of the perforant path. *The Journal of Physiology* **232**, 331–356, doi:10.1113/jphysiol.1973.sp010273 (1973).

35 Glanzman, D. L. Octopus conditioning: a multi-armed approach to the LTP–learning question. *Curr. Biol.* **18**, R527-R530, doi:dx.doi.org/10.1016/j.cub.2008.04.046 (2008).

36 Shomrat, T., Zarrella, I., Fiorito, G. & Hochner, B. The octopus vertical lobe modulates short-term learning rate and uses LTP to acquire long-term memory. *Curr. Biol.* **18**, 337–342, doi:dx.doi.org/10.1016/j.cub.2008.01.056 (2008).

37 Brown, E. R. & Piscopo, S. Synaptic plasticity in cephalopods; more than just learning and memory? *Invertebrate Neuroscience* **13**, 35–44, doi:10.1007/s10158-013-0150-4 (2013).

38 Burkhardt, P. The origin and evolution of synaptic proteins: choanoflagellates lead the way. *Journal of Experimental Biology* **218**, 506–514, doi:10.1242/jeb.110247 (2015).

39 Emes, R. D. & Grant, S. G. N. in *Annual Review of Neuroscience* **35** (ed. S. E. Hyman), 111–131 (Annual Reviews, 2012).

40 Kontra, C., Lyons, D. J., Fischer, S. M. & Beilock, S. L. Physical experience enhances science learning. *Psychological Science* **26**, 737–749, doi:10.1177/0956797615569355 (2015).

41 Toumpaniari, K., Loyens, S., Mavilidi, M.-F. & Paas, F. Preschool children's foreign language vocabulary learning by embodying words through physical activity and gesturing. *Educational Psychology Review* **27**, 445–456, doi:10.1007/s10648-015-9316-4 (2015).

42 Engelkamp, J., Seiler, K. & Zimmer, H. Memory for actions: item and relational information in categorized lists. *Psychological Research* **69**, 1–10, doi:10.1007/s00426-003-0160-7 (2004).

43 Agostinho, S. *et al.* Giving learning a helping hand: finger tracing of temperature graphs on an iPad. *Educational Psychology Review* **27**, 427–443, doi:10.1007/s10648-015-9315-5 (2015).

44 Ruiter, M., Loyens, S. & Paas, F. Watch your step children! Learning two-digit numbers through mirror-based observation of self-initiated body movements. *Educational Psychology Review* **27**, 457–474, doi:10.1007/s10648-015-9324-4 (2015).

45 Mason, P. R. Chemo-klino-kinesis in planarian food location. *Anim. Behav.* **23**, 460–469, doi:10.1016/0003-3472(75)90095-0 (1975).

46 Miyamoto, S. & Shimozawa, A. Chemotaxis in the fresh-water planarian, Dugesia-japonica-japonica. *Zoological Science* **2**, 389–395 (1985).

47 Brown, H. M. & Ogden, T. E. Electrical response of planarian ocellus. *Journal of General Physiology* **51**, 237, doi:10.1085/jgp.51.2.237 (1968).

48 Brown, F. A. Effects and after-effects on planarians of reversals of horizontal magnetic vector. *Nature* **209**, 533, doi:10.1038/209533b0 (1966).

49 Brown, F. A. & Chow, C. S. Differentiation between clockwise and counter-clockwise magnetic rotation by planarian, Dugesia dorotacephala. *Physiological Zoology* **48**, 168–176 (1975).

50 Sarnat, H. B. & Netsky, M. G. When does a ganglion become a brain? Evolutionary origin of the central nervous system. *Seminars in Pediatric Neurology* **9**, 240–253, doi:10.1053/spen.2002.32502 (2002).

51 Buttarelli, F. R., Pellicano, C. & Pontieri, F. E. Neuropharmacology and behavior in planarians: translations to mammals. *Comparative Biochemistry and Physiology C-Toxicology & Pharmacology* **147**, 399–408, doi:10.1016/j.cbpc.2008.01.009 (2008).

52 Ribeiro, P. & Patocka, N. Neurotransmitter transporters in schistosomes: structure, function and prospects for drug discovery. *Parasitol. Int.* **62**, 629–638, doi:10.1016/j.parint.2013.06.003 (2013).

53 Hagstrom, D., Cochet-Escartin, O., Zhang, S., Khuu, C. & Collins, E.-M. S. Freshwater planarians as an alternative animal model for neurotoxicology. *Toxicological Sciences* **147**, 270–285, doi:10.1093/toxsci/kfv129 (2015).

54 Wisenden, B. D. & Millard, M. C. Aquatic flatworms use chemical cues from injured conspecifics to assess predation risk and to associate risk with novel cues. *Anim. Behav.* **62**, 761–766, doi:10.1006/anbe.2001.1797 (2001).

55 Shomrat, T. & Levin, M. An automated training paradigm reveals long-term memory in planarians and its persistence through head regeneration. *Journal of Experimental Biology* **216**, 3799–3810, doi:10.1242/jeb.087809 (2013).

56 Yoon, H. S., Hackett, J. D., Ciniglia, C., Pinto, G. & Bhattacharya, D. A molecular timeline for the origin of photosynthetic eukaryotes. *Mol. Biol. Evol.* **21**, 809–818, doi:10.1093/molbev/msh075 (2004).

57 Keeling, P. J. The endosymbiotic origin, diversification and fate of plastids. *Philos. Trans. R. Soc. B-Biol. Sci.* **365**, 729–748, doi:10.1098/rstb.2009.0103 (2010).

58 Leliaert, F. *et al.* Phylogeny and molecular evolution of the green algae. *Crit. Rev. Plant Sci.* **31**, 1–46, doi:10.1080/07352689.2011.615705 (2012).

59 Hedges, S. B., Blair, J. E., Venturi, M. L. & Shoe, J. L. A molecular timescale of eukaryote evolution and the rise of complex multicellular life. *BMC Evol. Biol.* **4**, 9, doi:10.1186/1471-2148-4-2 (2004).

60 Wellman, C. H., Osterloff, P. L. & Mohiuddin, U. Fragments of the earliest land plants. *Nature* **425**, 282–285, doi:10.1038/nature01884 (2003).

61 Ahlberg, P. E., Smith, M. M. & Johanson, Z. Developmental plasticity and disparity in early dipnoan (lungfish) dentitions. *Evolution & Development* **8**, 331–349, doi:10.1111/j.1525-142X.2006.00106.x (2006).

62 Campbell, K. S. W. & Wragg, S. Structural details of Early Devonian dipnoans. *Australian Journal of Zoology* **62**, 18–25, doi:10.1071/zo13055 (2014).

63 Niedzwiedzki, G., Szrek, P., Narkiewicz, K., Narkiewicz, M. & Ahlberg, P. E. Tetrapod trackways from the early Middle Devonian period of Poland. *Nature* **463**, 43–48, doi:10.1038/nature08623 (2010).

64 Ahlberg, P. E. & Milner, A. R. The origin and early diversification of tetrapods. *Nature* **368**, 507–514, doi:10.1038/368507a0 (1994).

65 Janis, C. M. & Keller, J. C. Modes of ventilation in early tetrapods: costal aspiration as a key feature of amniotes. *Acta Palaeontol. Pol.* **46**, 137–170 (2001).

66 Clack, J. A. *Gaining ground: The origin and early evolution of tetrapods* (Indiana University Press, 2002).

67 Delfino, M. & Sanchez-Villagra, M. R. A survey of the rock record of reptilian ontogeny. *Semin. Cell Dev. Biol.* **21**, 432–440, doi:10.1016/j.semcdb.2009.11.007 (2010).

68 Adapted from G. Roth and U. Dicke. *Evolution of nervous systems and brains* (Springer, 2013).

69 Pearson, M. R., Benson, R. B. J., Upchurch, P., Fröbisch, J. & Kammerer, C. F. Reconstructing the diversity of early terrestrial herbivorous tetrapods. *Palaeogeography, Palaeoclimatology, Palaeoecology* **372**, 42–49, doi:dx.doi.org/10.1016/j.palaeo.2012.11.008 (2013).

70 Mink, J. W., Blumenschine, R. J. & Adams, D. B. Ratio of central nervous-system to body metabolism in vertebrates: its constancy and functional basis. *American Journal of Physiology* **241**, R203-R212 (1981).

71 Roth, G. & Dicke, U. Evolution of the brain and intelligence. *Trends in Cognitive Sciences* **9**, 250–257, doi:10.1016/j.tics.2005.03.005 (2005).

72 Kaas, J. H. *The thalamus revisited: Where do we go from here?* Vol. 130 (Oxford University Press, 2007).

73 Sarko, D. K., Rice, F. L. & Reep, R. L. in *New Perspectives on Neurobehavioral Evolution* **1225**, *Annals of the New York Academy of Sciences* (eds J. I. Johnson, H. P. Zeigler & P. R. Hof), 90–100 (2011).

74 Jacobs, L. F. From chemotaxis to the cognitive map: the function of olfaction. *Proc. Natl. Acad. Sci. U.S.A.* **109**, 10693–10700, doi:10.1073/pnas.1201880109 (2012).

75 Rowe, T. B., Macrini, T. E. & Luo, Z. X. Fossil evidence on origin of the mammalian brain. *Science* **332**, 955–957, doi:10.1126/science.1203117 (2011).

76 Dooley, J. C., Franca, J. G., Seelke, A. M. H., Cooke, D. F. & Krubitzer, L. A. Evolution of mammalian sensorimotor cortex: thalamic projections to parietal cortical areas in Monodelphis domestica. *Front. Neuroanat.* **8**, 21, doi:10.3389/fnana.2014.00163 (2015).

77 Ghahramani, Z. in *Advanced Lectures on Machine Learning*, Vol. 3176, *Lecture Notes in Artificial Intelligence* (eds O. Bousquet, U. VonLuxburg & G. Ratsch), 72–112 (Springer-Verlag, Berlin, 2004).

78 Jerison, H. J. Animal intelligence as encephalization. *Philos. Trans. R. Soc. Lond. Ser. B-Biol. Sci.* **308**, 21–35, doi:10.1098/rstb.1985.0007 (1985).

79 Nieuwenhuys, R. The neocortex: an overview of its evolutionary development, structural organization and synpatology. *Anatomy and Embryology* **190**, 307–337 (1994).

80 Kriegstein, A., Noctor, S. & Martinez-Cerdeno, V. Patterns of neural stem and progenitor cell division may underlie evolutionary cortical expansion. *Nature Reviews Neuroscience* **7**, 883–890, doi:10.1038/nrn2008 (2006).

81 Lui, J. H., Hansen, D. V. & Kriegstein, A. R. Development and evolution of the human neocortex. *Cell* **146**, 18–36, doi:10.1016/j.cell.2011.06.030 (2011).

82 DeFelipe, J. The evolution of the brain, the human nature of cortical circuits, and intellectual creativity. *Front. Neuroanat.* **5**, 17, doi:10.3389/fnana.2011.00029 (2011).

83 Raizada, R. D. S. & Grossberg, S. Towards a theory of the laminar architecture of cerebral cortex: computational clues from the visual system. *Cerebral Cortex* **13**, 100–113, doi:10.1093/cercor/13.1.100 (2003).

84 Miller, G. A. The magical number 7, plus or minus 2: some limits on our capacity for processing information. *Psychological Review* **63**, 81–97, doi:10.1037//0033-295x.101.2.343 (1956).

85 Curtis, C. E. & D'Esposito, M. Persistent activity in the prefrontal cortex during working memory. *Trends in Cognitive Sciences* **7**, 415–423 (2003).

86 Koziol, L. F. *et al.* Consensus paper: the cerebellum's role in movement and cognition. *The Cerebellum* **13**, 151–177, doi:10.1007/s12311-013-0511-x (2013).

87 Popa, L. S., Streng, M. L., Hewitt, A. L. & Ebner, T. J. The errors of our ways: understanding error representations in cerebellar-dependent motor learning. *Cerebellum* **15**, 93–103, doi:10.1007/s12311-015-0685-5 (2016).

88 Doya, K. Complementary roles of basal ganglia and cerebellum in learning and motor control. *Curr. Opin. Neurobiol.* **10**, 732–739, doi:10.1016/s0959-4388(00)00153-7 (2000).

89 Strick, P. L., Dum, R. P. & Fiez, J. A. in *Annual Review of Neuroscience* **32**, 413–434 (Annual Reviews, 2009).

90 Janvier, P. microRNAs revive old views about jawless vertebrate divergence and evolution. *Proc. Natl. Acad. Sci. U.S.A.* **107**, 19137–19138, doi:10.1073/pnas.1014583107 (2010).

91 Grillner, S. & Robertson, B. The basal ganglia downstream control of brainstem motor centres: an evolutionarily conserved strategy. *Curr. Opin. Neurobiol.* **33**, 47–52, doi:dx.doi.org/10.1016/j.conb.2015.01.019 (2015).

92 Grillner, S. & Robertson, B. The basal ganglia downstream control of brainstem motor centres: an evolutionarily conserved strategy. *Curr. Opin. Neurobiol.* **33**, 47–52, doi:dx.doi.org/10.1016/j.conb.2015.01.019 (2015).

93 Marin, O., Gonzalez, A. & Smeets, W. Basal ganglia organization in amphibians: afferent connections to the striatum and the nucleus accumbens. *Journal of Comparative Neurology* **378**, 16–49, doi:10.1002/(sici)1096-9861(19970203)378:1<16::aid-cne2>3.0.co;2-n (1997).

94 Skelin, I. *et al.* Lesions of dorsal striatum eliminate lose-switch responding but not mixed-response strategies in rats. *European Journal of Neuroscience* **39**, 1655–1663, doi:10.1111/ejn.12518 (2014).

95 Leblois, A., Wendel, B. J. & Perkel, D. J. Striatal dopamine modulates basal ganglia output and regulates social context-dependent behavioral variability through D-1 receptors. *Journal of Neuroscience* **30**, 5730–5743, doi:10.1523/jneurosci.5974-09.2010 (2010).

96 Daw, N. D., O'Doherty, J. P., Dayan, P., Seymour, B. & Dolan, R. J. Cortical substrates for exploratory decisions in humans. *Nature* **441**, 876–879, doi:10.1038/nature04766 (2006).

97 Horga, G. *et al.* Changes in corticostriatal connectivity during reinforcement learning in humans. *Human Brain Mapping* **36**, 793–803, doi:10.1002/hbm.22665 (2015).

98 Jacobs, L. F. The evolution of the cognitive map. *Brain Behav. Evol.* **62**, 128–139, doi:10.1159/000072443 (2003).

99 Allen, T. A. & Fortin, N. J. The evolution of episodic memory. *Proc. Natl. Acad. Sci. U.S.A.* **110**, 10379–10386, doi:10.1073/pnas.1301199110 (2013).

100 Tononi, G. & Cirelli, C. Sleep and the price of plasticity: from synaptic and cellular homeostasis to memory consolidation and integration. *Neuron* **81**, 12–34, doi:10.1016/j.neuron.2013.12.025 (2014).

101 Maquet, P. *et al.* Experience dependent changes in cerebral activation during human REM sleep. *Nature Neuroscience* **3**, 831–836 (2000).

102 Calamaro, C. J., Yang, K., Ratcliffe, S. & Chasens, E. R. Wired at a young age: the effect of caffeine and technology on sleep duration and body mass index in school-aged children. *J. Pediatr. Health Care* **26**, 276–282, doi:10.1016/j.pedhc.2010.12.002 (2012).

103 Dworak, M., Schierl, T., Bruns, T. & Struder, H. K. Impact of singular excessive computer game and television exposure on sleep patterns and memory performance of school-aged children. *Pediatrics* **120**, 978–985, doi:10.1542/peds.2007-0476 (2007).

104 Jackson, C. *et al.* Dynamic effects of a memory trace: sleep on consolidation. *Curr. Biol.* **18**, 393–400, doi:10.1016/j.cub.2008.01.062 (2008).

105 Vorster, A. P. & Born, J. Sleep and memory in mammals, birds and invertebrates. *Neurosci. Biobehav. Rev.* **50**, 103–119, doi:10.1016/j.neubiorev.2014.09.020 (2015).

106 Beyaert, L., Greggers, U. & Menzel, R. Honeybees consolidate navigation memory during sleep. *Journal of Experimental Biology* **215**, 3981–3988, doi:10.1242/jeb.075499 (2012).

107 Tononi, G. & Cirelli, C. Steep function and synaptic homeostasis. *Sleep Medicine Reviews* **10**, 49–62, doi:10.1016/j.smrv.2005.05.002 (2006).

108 Bushey, D., Tononi, G. & Cirelli, C. Sleep- and wake-dependent changes in neuronal activity and reactivity demonstrated in fly neurons using in vivo calcium imaging. *Proc. Natl. Acad. Sci. U.S.A.* **112**, 4785–4790, doi:10.1073/pnas.1419603112 (2015).

109 Kirszenblat, L. & van Swinderen, B. The yin and yang of sleep and attention. *Trends in Neurosciences* **38**, 776–786, doi:dx.doi.org/10.1016/j.tins.2015.10.001 (2015).

110 Cho, J. Y. & Sternberg, P. W. Multilevel modulation of a sensory motor circuit during C. elegans sleep and arousal. *Cell* **156**, 249–260, doi:10.1016/j.cell.2013.11.036 (2014).

111 Papini, M. R. Comparative psychology of surprising nonreward. *Brain Behav. Evol.* **62**, 83–95, doi:10.1159/000072439 (2003).

112 Thaker, M., Vanak, A. T., Lima, S. L. & Hews, D. K. Stress and aversive learning in a wild vertebrate: the role of corticosterone in mediating escape from a novel stressor. *Am. Nat.* **175**, 50–60, doi:10.1086/648558 (2010).

113 Overmier, J. B. & Papini, M. R. Factors modulating the effects of teleost telencephalon ablation on retention, relearning and extinction of instrumental avoidance behavior. *Behav. Neurosci.* **100**, 190, doi:10.1037/0735-7044.100.2.190 (1986).

114 Portavella, M., Salas, C., Vargas, J. P. & Papini, M. R. Involvement of the telencephalon in spaced-trial avoidance learning in the goldfish (Carassius auratus). *Physiol. Behav.* **80**, 49–56, doi:10.1016/s0031-9384(03)00208-7 (2003).

115 Portavella, M., Torres, B. & Salas, C. Avoidance response in goldfish: emotional and temporal involvement of medial and lateral telencephalic pallium. *Journal of Neuroscience* **24**, 2335–2342, doi:10.1523/jneurosci.4930-03.2004 (2004).

116 Laberge, F., Muhlenbrock-Lenter, S., Grunwald, W. & Roth, G. Evolution of the amygdala: new insights from studies in amphibians. *Brain Behav. Evol.* **67**, 177–187, doi:10.1159/000091119 (2006).

117 Bitterman, M. E. Comparative analysis of learning: are laws of learning same in all animals? *Science* **188**, 699–709, doi:10.1126/science.188.4189.699 (1975).

118 Schwabe, L., Joels, M., Roozendaal, B., Wolf, O. T. & Oitzl, M. S. Stress effects on memory: an update and integration. *Neurosci. Biobehav. Rev.* **36**, 1740–1749, doi:10.1016/j.neubiorev.2011.07.002 (2012).

119 Kromann, C. B., Jensen, M. L. & Ringsted, C. Test-enhanced learning may be a gender-related phenomenon explained by changes in cortisol level. *Medical Education* **45**, 192–199, doi:10.1111/j.1365-2923.2010.03790.x (2011).

120 Lee, H., Park, J., Kim, S. & Han, J. Cortisol as a predictor of simulation-based educational outcomes in senior nursing students: a pilot study. *Clinical Simulation in Nursing* **12**, 44–48, doi:10.1016/j.ecns.2015.12.008 (2016).

121 Joels, M., Pu, Z. W., Wiegert, O., Oitzl, M. S. & Krugers, H. J. Learning under stress: how does it work? *Trends in Cognitive Sciences* **10**, 152–158 (2006).

122 Adapted from Schwabe, L. Stress effects on memory: an update and integration. *Neurosci. Biobehav. Rev.* **36**, 7, 1740–1749 (2012). doi: 10.1016/j.neubiorev.2011.07.002.

123 Roozendaal, B., McEwen, B. S. & Chattarji, S. Stress, memory and the amygdala. *Nature Reviews Neuroscience* **10**, 423–433, doi:10.1038/nrn2651 (2009).

124 Young, C. B., Wu, S. S. & Menon, V. The neurodevelopmental basis of math anxiety. *Psychological Science* **23**, 492–501, doi:10.1177/0956797611429134 (2012).

125 Hunter, A. L., Minnis, H. & Wilson, P. Altered stress responses in children exposed to early adversity: a systematic review of salivary cortisol studies. *Stress: The International Journal on the Biology of Stress* **14**, 614–626, doi:10.3109/10253890.2011.577848 (2011).

126 Hart, H. & Rubia, K. Neuroimaging of child abuse: a critical review. *Front. Hum. Neurosci.* **6**, 24, doi:10.3389/fnhum.2012.00052 (2012).

127 Bostan, A. C., Dum, R. P. & Strick, P. L. Cerebellar networks with the cerebral cortex and basal ganglia. *Trends in Cognitive Sciences* **17**, 241–254, doi:10.1016/j.tics.2013.03.003 (2013).

128 Adcock, R. A. Reward-motivated learning: mesolimbic activation precedes memory formation. *Neuron* **50**, 507–517 (2006).

129 Kikuchi, R. & Vanneste, M. A theoretical exercise in the modeling of ground-level ozone resulting from the K-T asteroid impact: its possible link with the extinction selectivity of terrestrial vertebrates. *Palaeogeography Palaeoclimatology Palaeoecology* **288**, 14–23, doi:10.1016/j.palaeo.2010.01.027 (2010).

130 Robertson, D. S., McKenna, M. C., Toon, O. B., Hope, S. & Lillegraven, J. A. Survival in the first hours of the Cenozoic. *Geological Society of America Bulletin* **116**, 760–768, doi:10.1130/b25402.1 (2004).

131 Howard-Jones, P. A., Demetriou, S., Bogacz, R., Yoo, J. H. & Leonards, U. Toward a science of learning games. *Mind, Brain, and Education* **5**, 33–41 (2011).

132 Callan, D. E. & Schweighofer, N. Positive and negative modulation of word learning by reward anticipation. *Human Brain Mapping* **29**, 237–249, doi:10.1002/hbm.20383 (2008).

133 Schultz, W., Dayan, P. & Montague, P. R. A neural substrate of prediction and reward. *Science* **275**, 1593–1599 (1997).

134 Nieuwenhuis, S. *et al.* Activity in human reward-sensitive brain areas is strongly context dependent. *Neuroimage* **25**, 1302–1309 (2005).

135 Steinberg, L. A behavioral scientist looks at the science of adolescent brain development. *Brain and Cognition* **72**, 160–164, doi:10.1016/j.bandc.2009.11.003 (2010).

136 Fiorillo, C. D., Tobler, P. N. & Schultz, W. Discrete coding of reward probability and uncertainty by dopamine neurons. *Science* **299**, 1898–1902 (2003).

137 Devonshire, I. M. *et al.* Risk-based learning games improve long-term retention of information among school pupils. *PLoS ONE* **9**, e103640 (2014).

138 Ozcelik, E., Cagiltay, N. E. & Ozcelik, N. S. The effect of uncertainty on learning in game-like environments. *Computers & Education* **67**, 12–20, doi:dx.doi.org/10.1016/j.compedu.2013.02.009 (2013).

139 Feduccia, A. Avian extinction at the end of the Cretaceous: assessing the magnitude and subsequent explosive radiation. *Cretac. Res.* **50**, 1–15, doi:10.1016/j.cretres.2014.03.009 (2014).

140 Jablonski, D. & Chaloner, W. G. Extinctions in the fossil record. *Philos. Trans. R. Soc. Lond. Ser. B-Biol. Sci.* **344**, 11–16, doi:10.1098/rstb.1994.0045 (1994).

141 Janzen, D. H. Who survived the cretaceous? *Science* **268**, 785, doi:10.1126/science.268.5212.785-a (1995).

142 Zachos, J. C., Dickens, G. R. & Zeebe, R. E. An early Cenozoic perspective on greenhouse warming and carbon-cycle dynamics. *Nature* **451**, 279–283, doi:10.1038/nature06588 (2008).

143 Dickens, G. R. Rethinking the global carbon cycle with a large, dynamic and microbially mediated gas hydrate capacitor. *Earth and Planetary Science Letters* **213**, 169–183, doi:dx.doi.org/10.1016/S0012-821X(03)00325-X (2003).

144 Chester, S. G. B., Bloch, J. I., Boyer, D. M. & Clemens, W. A. Oldest known euarchontan tarsals and affinities of Paleocene Purgatorius to primates. *Proc. Natl. Acad. Sci. U.S.A.* **112**, 1487–1492, doi:10.1073/pnas.1421707112 (2015).

145 Adapted from Orliac *et al.*, Endocranial morphology of Palaeocene Plesiadapis tricuspidens and evolution of the early primate brain. *Proc. Biol. Sci.* **281**, 1781, (2014).

146 Cartmill, M. Rethinking primate origins. *Science* **184**, 436–443, doi:10.1126/science.184.4135.436 (1974).

147 Sussman, R. W., Rasmussen, D. T. & Raven, P. H. Rethinking primate origins again. *American Journal of Primatology* **75**, 95–106, doi:10.1002/ajp.22096 (2013).

148 Herculano-Houzel, S., Collins, C. E., Wong, P. Y. & Kaas, J. H. Cellular scaling rules for primate brains. *Proc. Natl. Acad. Sci. U.S.A.* **104**, 3562–3567, doi:10.1073/pnas.0611396104 (2007).

149 Whishaw, I. Q. & Karl, J. M. The contribution of the reach and the grasp to shaping brain and behaviour. *Can. J. Exp. Psychol.-Rev. Can. Psychol. Exp.* **68**, 223–235, doi:10.1037/cep0000042 (2014).

150 Collins, C. E., Airey, D. C., Young, N. A., Leitch, D. B. & Kaas, J. H. Neuron densities vary across and within cortical areas in primates. *Proc. Natl. Acad. Sci. U.S.A.* **107**, 15927–15932, doi:10.1073/pnas.1010356107 (2010).

151 Begun, D. R. in *Annual Review of Anthropology* **39** (eds D. Brenneis & P. T. Ellison), 67–84 (Annual Reviews, 2010).

152 Nakatsukasa, M. *et al.* Definitive evidence for tail loss in Nacholapithecus, an East African Miocene hominoid. *J. Hum. Evol.* **45**, 179–186, doi:dx.doi.org/10.1016/S0047-2484(03)00092-7 (2003).

153 Begun, D. R., Nargolwalla, M. C. & Kordos, L. European miocene hominids and the origin of the African ape and human clade. *Evol. Anthropol.* **21**, 10–23, doi:10.1002/evan.20329 (2012).

154 Stewart, C. B. & Disotell, T. R. Primate evolution: in and out of Africa. *Curr. Biol.* **8**, R582-R588, doi:10.1016/s0960-9822(07)00367-3 (1998).

155 Wood, B. & Harrison, T. The evolutionary context of the first hominins. *Nature* **470**, 347–352 (2011).

156 Abernethy, K. A., White, L. J. T. & Wickings, E. J. Hordes of mandrills (Mandrillus sphinx): extreme group size and seasonal male presence. *Journal of Zoology* **258**, 131–137, doi:10.1017/s0952836902001267 (2002).

157 Hamilton, W. D. Geometry for selfish herd. *Journal of Theoretical Biology* **31**, 295, doi:10.1016/0022-5193(71)90189-5 (1971).

158 Wrangham, R. W. An ecological model of female-bonded primate groups. *Behaviour* **75**, 262–300, doi:10.1163/156853980x00447 (1980).

159 Dunbar, R. I. M. & Shultz, S. Evolution in the social brain. *Science* **317**, 1344–1347, doi:10.1126/science.1145463 (2007).

160 Dunbar, R. I. M. Coevolution of neocortical size, group size and language in humans. *Behav. Brain Sci.* **16**, 681–735 (1993).

161 Hill, R. A. & Dunbar, R. I. M. Social network size in humans. *Hum. Nat.-Interdiscip. Biosoc. Perspect.* **14**, 53–72, doi:10.1007/s12110-003-1016-y (2003).

162 Roberts, S. G. B., Dunbar, R. I. M., Pollet, T. V. & Kuppens, T. Exploring variation in active network size: constraints and ego characteristics. *Social Networks* **31**, 138–146, doi:dx.doi.org/10.1016/j.socnet.2008.12.002 (2009).

163 Dunbar, R. I. M., Arnaboldi, V., Conti, M. & Passarella, A. The structure of online social networks mirrors those in the offline world. *Social Networks* **43**, 39–47, doi:10.1016/j.socnet.2015.04.005 (2015).

164 Kanai, R., Bahrami, B., Roylance, R. & Rees, G. Online social network size is reflected in human brain structure. *Proc. R. Soc. B-Biol. Sci.* **279**, 1327–1334, doi:10.1098/rspb.2011.1959 (2012).

165 Herculano-Houzel, S., Manger, P. R. & Kaas, J. H. Brain scaling in mammalian evolution as a consequence of concerted and mosaic changes in numbers of neurons and average neuronal cell size. *Front. Neuroanat.* **8**, doi:10.3389/fnana.2014.00077 (2014).

166 Herculano-Houzel, S., Manger, P. R. & Kaas, J. H. Brain scaling in mammalian evolution as a consequence of concerted and mosaic changes in numbers of neurons and average neuronal cell size. *Front. Neuroanat.* **8**, doi:10.3389/fnana.2014.00077 (2014).

167 Herculano-Houzel, S. The human brain in numbers: a linearly scaled-up primate brain. *Front. Hum. Neurosci.* **3**, doi:10.3389/neuro.09.031.2009 (2009).

168 van Schaik, C. P., Isler, K. & Burkart, J. M. Explaining brain size variation: from social to cultural brain. *Trends in Cognitive Sciences* **16**, 277–284, doi:10.1016/j.tics.2012.04.004 (2012).

169 Grueter, C. C. Home range overlap as a driver of intelligence in primates. *American Journal of Primatology* **77**, 418–424, doi:10.1002/ajp.22357 (2015).

170 Burkart, J. M. & Finkenwirth, C. Marmosets as model species in neuroscience and evolutionary anthropology. *Neuroscience Research* **93**, 8–19, doi:dx.doi.org/10.1016/j.neures.2014.09.003 (2015).

171 Clay, Z. & de Waal, F. B. M. Bonobos respond to distress in others: consolation across the age spectrum. *PLoS ONE* **8**, e55206, doi:10.1371/journal.pone.0055206 (2013).

172 Goodall, J. *Through a window: My thirty years with the chimpanzees of Gombe* (Houghton Mifflin, 1990).

173 Cheney, D. L. & Seyfarth, R. M. Vocal recognition in free-ranging vervet monkeys. *Anim. Behav.* **28**, 362-367, doi:10.1016/s0003-3472(80)80044-3 (1980).

174 Massen, J. J. M., Pasukonis, A., Schmidt, J. & Bugnyar, T. Ravens notice dominance reversals among conspecifics within and outside their social group. *Nature Communications* **5**, 7, doi:10.1038/ncomms4679 (2014).

175 Schulke, O., Bhagavatula, J., Vigilant, L. & Ostner, J. Social bonds enhance reproductive success in male macaques. *Curr. Biol.* **20**, 2207–2210, doi:10.1016/j.cub.2010.10.058 (2010).

176 de Waal, F. *Chimpanzee politics: Sex and power among apes* (Johns Hopkins University Press, 1982).

177 Nishida, T. & Hosaka, K. *Coalition strategies among adult male chimpanzees of the Mahale Mountains, Tanzania* (Cambridge University Press, 1996).

178 Nishida, T. Alpha status and agonistic alliance in wild chimpanzees pan-troglodytes-schweinfurthii. *Primates* **24**, 318–336, doi:10.1007/bf02381978 (1983).

179 Bissonnette, A., Franz, M., Schulke, O. & Ostner, J. Socioecology, but not cognition, predicts male coalitions across primates. *Behavioral Ecology* **25**, 794–801, doi:10.1093/beheco/aru054 (2014).

180 Higham, J. P. & Maestripieri, D. Revolutionary coalitions in male rhesus macaques. *Behaviour* **147**, 1889–1908, doi:10.1163/000579510x539709 (2010).

181 Tomasello, M. & Call, J. *Primate cognition* (Oxford University Press, 1997).

182 Call, J. & Tomasello, M. Does the chimpanzee have a theory of mind? 30 years later. *Trends in Cognitive Sciences* **12**, 187–192, doi:10.1016/j.tics.2008.02.010 (2008).

183 Kaminski, J., Call, J. & Tomasello, M. Body orientation and face orientation: two factors controlling apes' begging behavior from humans. *Anim. Cogn.* **7**, 216–223, doi:10.1007/s10071-004-0214-2 (2004).

184 Liebal, K., Pika, S., Call, J. & Tomasello, M. To move or not to move: how apes adjust to the attentional state of others. *Interact. Stud.* **5**, 199–219, doi:10.1075/is.5.2.03lie (2004).

185 Hare, B., Call, J. & Tomasello, M. Do chimpanzees know what conspecifics know? *Anim. Behav.* **61**, 139–151, doi:10.1006/anbe.2000.1518 (2001).

186 Kaminski, J., Call, J. & Tomasello, M. Chimpanzees know what others know, but not what they believe. *Cognition* **109**, 224–234, doi:10.1016/j.cognition.2008.08.010 (2008).

187 Flombaum, J. I. & Santos, L. R. Rhesus monkeys attribute perceptions to others. *Curr. Biol.* **15**, 447–452, doi:10.1016/j.cub.2004.12.076 (2005).

188 Santos, L. R., Nissen, A. G. & Ferrugia, J. A. Rhesus monkeys, Macaca mulatta, know what others can and cannot hear. *Anim. Behav.* **71**, 1175–1181, doi:10.1016/j.anbehav.2005.10.007 (2006).

189 Karg, K., Schmelz, M., Call, J. & Tomasello, M. The goggles experiment: can chimpanzees use self-experience to infer what a competitor can see? *Anim. Behav.* **105**, 211–221, doi:10.1016/j.anbehav.2015.04.028 (2015).

190 Krupenye, C., Kano, F., Hirata, S., Call, J. & Tomasello, M. Great apes anticipate that other individuals will act according to false beliefs. *Science* **354**, 110–114, doi:10.1126/science.aaf8110 (2016).

191 Heyes, C. Grist and mills: on the cultural origins of cultural learning. *Philos. Trans. R. Soc. B-Biol. Sci.* **367**, 2181–2191, doi:10.1098/rstb.2012.0120 (2012).

192 Gariepy, J. F. *et al.* Social learning in humans and other animals. *Frontiers in Neuroscience* **8**, 13, doi:10.3389/fnins.2014.00058 (2014).

193 Shimpi, P. M., Akhtar, N. & Moore, C. Toddlers' imitative learning in inter-active and observational contexts: the role of age and familiarity of the model. *J. Exp. Child Psychol.* **116**, 309–323, doi:10.1016/j.jecp.2013.06.008 (2013).

194 Ledford, J. R. & Wolery, M. Observational learning of academic and social behaviors during small-group direct instruction. *Exceptional Children* **81**, 272–291, doi:10.1177/0014402914563698 (2015).

195 Birch, L. L. Effects of peer models' food choices and eating behaviours on preschoolers' food preferences. *Child Development* **51**, 489–496, doi:10.2307/1129283 (1980).

196 Ste-Marie, D. M. *et al.* Observation interventions for motor skill learning and performance: an applied model for the use of observation. *International Review of Sport and Exercise Psychology* **5**, 145–176, doi:10.1080/17509 84X.2012.665076 (2012).

197 Olsson, A. & Phelps, E. A. Social learning of fear. *Nature Neuroscience* **10**, 1095–1102, doi:10.1038/nn1968 (2007).

198 Keller, M., Perrin, G., Meurisse, M., Ferreira, G. & Levy, F. Cortical and medial amygdala are both involved in the formation of olfactory offspring memory in sheep. *European Journal of Neuroscience* **20**, 3433–3441, doi:10.1111/j.1460-9568.2004.03812.x (2004).

199 Kavaliers, M., Choleris, E. & Colwell, D. D. Learning from others to cope with biting flies: social learning of fear-induced conditioned analgesia and active avoidance. *Behavioral Neuroscience* **115**, 661–674, doi:10.1037//0735-7044. 115.3.661 (2001).

200 John, E. R., Chesler, P., Bartlett, F. & Victor, I. Observation learning in cats. *Science* **159**, 1489, doi:10.1126/science.159.3822.1489 (1968).

201 Cook, M. & Mineka, S. Observational conditioning of fear to fear-relevant versus fear-irrelevant stimuli in rhesus-monkeys. *J. Abnorm. Psychol.* **98**, 448–459, doi:10.1037/0021-843x.98.4.448 (1989).

202 Jeon, D. *et al.* Observational fear learning involves affective pain system and Ca(v)1.2 Ca2+ channels in ACC. *Nature Neuroscience* **13**, 482–488, doi:10.1038/nn.2504 (2010).

203 Avery, M. L. Finding good food and avoiding bad food: does it help to associate with experienced flockmates? *Anim. Behav.* **48**, 1371–1378, doi:10.1006/anbe.1994.1373 (1994).

204 Brown, C. R. Cliff swallow colonies as information-centers. *Science* **234**, 83–85, doi:10.1126/science.234.4772.83 (1986).

205 Krebs, J. R. & Inman, A. J. Learning and foraging: individuals, groups and populations. *Am. Nat.* **140**, S63-S84, doi:10.1086/285397 (1992).

206 Krebs, J. R., Macroberts, M. H. & Cullen, J. M. Flocking and feeding in Great Tit Parus-Major: experimental study. *Ibis* **114**, 507, doi:10.1111/j.1474-919X.1972.tb00852.x (1972).

207 Spence, K. W. Experimental studies of learning and the higher mental processes in infra-human primates. *Psychological Bulletin* **34**, 806–850, doi:10.1037/h0061498 (1937).

208 Hikami, K., Hasegawa, Y. & Matsuzawa, T. Social transmission of food preferences in Japanese monkeys (Macaca-Fuscata) after mere exposure or aversion training. *J. Comp. Psychol.* **104**, 233–237, doi:10.1037//0735-7036.104.3.233 (1990).

209 Masuda, A. & Aou, S. Social transmission of avoidance behavior under situational change in learned and unlearned rats. *PLOS One* **4**, 7, doi:10.1371/journal.pone.0006794 (2009).

210 Patrick, H. & Nicklas, T. A. A review of family and social determinants of children's eating patterns and diet quality. *J. Am. Coll. Nutr.* **24**, 83–92 (2005).

211 Young, M. E., Mizzau, M., Mai, N. T., Sirisegaram, A. & Wilson, M. Food for thought: what you eat depends on your sex and eating companions. *Appetite* **53**, 268–271, doi:10.1016/j.appet.2009.07.021 (2009).

212 Sherry, D. F. & Galef, B. G. Cultural transmission without imitation: milk bottle opening by birds. *Anim. Behav.* **32**, 937–938, doi:10.1016/s0003-3472(84)80185-2 (1984).

213 Fiorito, G. & Scotto, P. Observational learning in Octopus Vulgaris. *Science* **256**, 545–547, doi:10.1126/science.256.5056.545 (1992).

214 Thornton, A. Social learning about novel foods in young meerkats. *Anim. Behav.* **76**, 1411–1421, doi:10.1016/j.anbehav.2008.07.007 (2008).

215 Itani, J. & Nishimura, A. in *Precultural primate behavior* (ed. E. W. Menzel), 26–50 (Karger, 1973).

216 Kawai, M. Newly acquired pre-cultural behavior of the natural troop of Japanese monkeys on Koshima Islet. *Primates* **6**, 1–30 (1965).

217 Kawamura, S. The process of sub-culture propagation amongst Japanese macaques. *Primates* **2**, 43–60 (1959).

218 Whiten, A. The scope of culture in chimpanzees, humans and ancestral apes. *Philosophical Transactions of the Royal Society B: Biological Sciences* **366**, 997–1007, doi:10.1098/rstb.2010.0334 (2011).

219 So, W. C., Chen-Hui, C. S. & Wei-Shan, J. L. Mnemonic effect of iconic gesture and beat gesture in adults and children: is meaning in gesture important for memory recall? *Language and Cognitive Processes* **27**, 665–681, doi:10.1080/01690965.2011.573220 (2012).

220 van Gog, T., Paas, F., Marcus, N., Ayres, P. & Sweller, J. The mirror neuron system and observational learning: implications for the effectiveness of dynamic learning. *Educational Psychology Review* **21**, 21–30 (2008).

221 Park, O. C. & Hopkins, R. Instructional conditions for using dynamic visual displays: a review. *Instructional Science* **21**, 427–449, doi:10.1007/bf00118557 (1993).

222 Wong, A. *et al.* Instructional animations can be superior to statics when learning human motor skills. *Computers in Human Behavior* **25**, 339–347, doi:10.1016/j.chb.2008.12.012 (2009).

223 Arguel, A. & Jamet, E. Using video and static pictures to improve learning of procedural contents. *Computers in Human Behavior* **25**, 354–359, doi:10.1016/j.chb.2008.12.014 (2009).

224 Ayres, P., Marcus, N., Chan, C. & Qian, N. X. Learning hand manipulative tasks: when instructional animations are superior to equivalent static representations. *Computers in Human Behavior* **25**, 348–353, doi:10.1016/j.chb.2008.12.013 (2009).

225 Wetzel, C. D., Radtke, P. H. & Stern, H. W. *Instructional effectiveness of video media* (Erlbaum, 1994).

226 Ayres, P. & Paas, F. Making instructional animations more effective: a cognitive load approach. *Appl. Cogn. Psychol.* **21**, 695–700, doi:10.1002/acp.1343 (2007).

227 Rizzolatti, G., Cattaneo, L., Fabbri-Destro, M. & Rozzi, S. Cortical mechanisms underlying the organization of goal-directed actions and mirror neuron-based action understanding. *Physiological Reviews* **94**, 655–706, doi:10.1152/physrev. 00009.2013 (2014).

228 Swaney, W., Kendal, J., Capon, H., Brown, C. & Laland, K. N. Familiarity facilitates social learning of foraging behaviour in the guppy. *Anim. Behav.* **62**, 591–598, doi:10.1006/anbe.2001.1788 (2001).

229 Nicol, C. How animals learn from each other. *Appl. Anim. Behav. Sci.* **100**, 58–63, doi:10.1016/j.applanim.2006.04.004 (2006).

230 Henrich, J. & Broesch, J. On the nature of cultural transmission networks: evidence from Fijian villages for adaptive learning biases. *Philos. Trans. R. Soc. B-Biol. Sci.* **366**, 1139–1148, doi:10.1098/rstb.2010.0323 (2011).

231 Menzel, E. W. in *Behavior of Non-human Primates: Modern Research Trends*, Vol. 5 (eds A. M. Schrier & F. Stollnitz), 93–153 (Academic Press, 1974).

232 Galef, B. G. & Laland, K. N. Social learning in animals: empirical studies and theoretical models. *Bioscience* **55**, 489–499, doi:10.1641/0006-3568(2005)055[0489:sliaes]2.0.co;2 (2005).

233 Behrens, T. E. J., Hunt, L. T., Woolrich, M. W. & Rushworth, M. F. S. Associative learning of social value. *Nature* **456**, 245–249, doi:10.1038/nature07538 (2008).

234 Deaner, R. O., Isler, K., Burkart, J. & van Schaik, C. Overall brain size, and not encephalization quotient, best predicts cognitive ability across non-human primates. *Brain Behav. Evol.* **70**, 115–124, doi:10.1159/000102973 (2007).

235 Reader, S. M., Hager, Y. & Laland, K. N. The evolution of primate general and cultural intelligence. *Philos. Trans. R. Soc. B-Biol. Sci.* **366**, 1017–1027, doi:10.1098/rstb.2010.0342 (2011).

236 Reader, S. M. & Laland, K. N. Social intelligence, innovation, and enhanced brain size in primates. *Proc. Natl. Acad. Sci. U.S.A.* **99**, 4436–4441, doi:10.1073/pnas.062041299 (2002).

237 Deaner, R. O., van Schaik, C. P. & Johnson, V. Do some taxa have better domain-general cognition than others? A meta-analysis of nonhuman primate studies. *Evolutionary Psychology* **4**, doi:10.1177/147470490600400114 (2006).

238 Marcovitch, S. & Zelazo, P. D. The A-not-B error: results from a logistic meta-analysis. *Child Development* **70**, 1297–1313, doi:10.1111/1467-8624.00095 (1999).

239 Piaget, J. *The construction of reality in the child* (Ballantine Books, 1954).

240 Barth, J. & Call, J. Tracking the displacement of objects: a series of tasks with great apes (Pan troglodytes, Pan paniscus, Gorilla gorilla, and Pongo pygmaeus) and young children (Homo sapiens). *J. Exp. Psychol.-Anim. Behav. Process.* **32**, 239–252, doi:10.1037/0097-7403.32.3.239 (2006).

241 Herrmann, E., Call, J., Hernandez-Lloreda, M. V., Hare, B. & Tomasello, M. Humans have evolved specialized skills of social cognition: the cultural intelligence hypothesis. *Science* **317**, 1360–1366, doi:10.1126/science.1146282 (2007).

242 Beran, M. J. Chimpanzees (Pan troglodytes) accurately compare poured liquid quantities. *Anim. Cogn.* **13**, 641–649, doi:10.1007/s10071-010-0314-0 (2010).

243 Beran, M. J. Monkeys (Macaca mulatta and Cebus apella) track, enumerate, and compare multiple sets of moving items. *J. Exp. Psychol.-Anim. Behav. Process.* **34**, 63–74, doi:10.1037/0097-7403.34.1.63 (2008).

244 Suda, C. & Call, J. Piagetian conservation of discrete quantities in bonobos (Pan paniscus), chimpanzees (Pan trogiodytes), and orangutans (Pongo pygmaeus). *Anim. Cogn.* **8**, 220–235, doi:10.1007/s10071-004-0247-6 (2005).

245 Piaget, J. *The child's conception of number* (W. Norton Company & Inc., 1965).

246 Furuichi, T. *et al.* Why do wild bonobos not use tools like chimpanzees do? *Behaviour* **152**, 425–460, doi:10.1163/1568539x-00003226 (2015).

247 Mendes, F. D. C. *et al.* Diversity of nutcracking tool sites used by Sapajus libidinosus in Brazilian Cerrado. *American Journal of Primatology* **77**, 535–546, doi:10.1002/ajp.22373 (2015).

248 Hanus, D. & Call, J. Chimpanzees infer the location of a reward on the basis of the effect of its weight. *Curr. Biol.* **18**, R370-R372, doi:10.1016/j.cub.2008.02.039 (2008).

249 Suddendorf, T. & Corballis, M. C. New evidence for animal foresight? *Anim. Behav.* **75**, E1–E3, doi:10.1016/j.anbehav.2008.01.006 (2008).

250 Mulcahy, N. J. & Call, J. Apes save tools for future use. *Science* **312**, 1038–1040, doi:10.1126/science.1125456 (2006).

251 Osvath, M. & Osvath, H. Chimpanzee (Pan troglodytes) and orangutan (Pongo abelii) forethought: self-control and pre-experience in the face of future tool use. *Anim. Cogn.* **11**, 661–674, doi:10.1007/s10071-008-0157-0 (2008).

252 Corti, G. Continental rift evolution: from rift initiation to incipient break-up in the Main Ethiopian Rift, East Africa. *Earth-Science Reviews* **96**, 1–53, doi:dx.doi.org/10.1016/j.earscirev.2009.06.005 (2009).

253 Sepulchre, P. *et al.* Tectonic uplift and Eastern Africa aridification. *Science* **313**, 1419–1423, doi:10.1126/science.1129158 (2006).

254 Trauth, M. H., Maslin, M. A., Deino, A. & Strecker, M. R. Late Cenozoic moisture history of East Africa. *Science* **309**, 2051–2053, doi:10.1126/science.1112964 (2005).

255 Cerling, T. E. *et al.* Global vegetation change through the Miocene/Pliocene boundary. *Nature* **389**, 153–158, doi:10.1038/38229 (1997).

256 Patterson, N., Richter, D. J., Gnerre, S., Lander, E. S. & Reich, D. Genetic evidence for complex speciation of humans and chimpanzees. *Nature* **441**, 1103–1108, doi:10.1038/nature04789 (2006).

257 Langergraber, K. E. *et al.* Generation times in wild chimpanzees and gorillas suggest earlier divergence times in great ape and human evolution. *Proc. Natl. Acad. Sci. U.S.A.* **109**, 15716–15721, doi:10.1073/pnas.1211740109 (2012).

258 Lebatard, A. E. *et al.* Cosmogenic nuclide dating of Sahelanthropus tchadensis and Australopithecus bahrelghazali: Mio-Pliocene hominids from Chad. *Proc. Natl. Acad. Sci. U.S.A.* **105**, 3226–3231, doi:10.1073/pnas.0708015105 (2008).

259 Brunet, M. *et al.* A new hominid from the Upper Miocene of Chad, Central Africa. *Nature* **418**, 145–151 (2002).

260 Wood, B. *Human evolution: A very short introduction* (Oxford University Press, 2005).

261 Senut, B. *et al.* First hominid from the Miocene (Lukeino Formation, Kenya). *Comptes Rendus De L Academie Des Sciences Serie Ii Fascicule a-Sciences De La Terre Et Des Planetes* **332**, 137–144, doi:10.1016/s1251-8050(01)01529-4 (2001).

262 Hublin, J. J. Paleoanthropology: how old is the oldest human? *Curr. Biol.* **25**, R453-R455, doi:10.1016/j.cub.2015.04.009 (2015).

263 Anton, S. C., Potts, R. & Aiello, L. C. Evolution of early Homo: an integrated biological perspective. *Science* **345**, 45, doi:10.1126/science.1236828 (2014).

264 Leakey, M. G. *et al.* New fossils from Koobi Fora in northern Kenya confirm taxonomic diversity in early Homo. *Nature* **488**, 201–204, doi:10.1038/nature11322 (2012).

265 Roach, N. T., Venkadesan, M., Rainbow, M. J. & Lieberman, D. E. Elastic energy storage in the shoulder and the evolution of high-speed throwing in Homo. *Nature* **498**, 483, doi:10.1038/nature12267 (2013).

266 Bramble, D. M. & Lieberman, D. E. Endurance running and the evolution of Homo. *Nature* **432**, 345–352, doi:10.1038/nature03052 (2004).

267 Ungar, P. S. Dental evidence for the reconstruction of diet in African early Homo. *Curr. Anthropol.* **53**, S318–S329, doi:10.1086/666700 (2012).

268 Maslin, M. A., Shultz, S. & Trauth, M. H. A synthesis of the theories and concepts of early human evolution. *Philos. Trans. R. Soc. B-Biol. Sci.* **370**, 12, doi:10.1098/rstb.2014.0064 (2015).

269 Wood, B. Fifty years after Homo habilis. *Nature* **508**, 31–33 (2014).

270 Levin, N. E. Environment and climate of early human evolution. *Annual Review of Earth and Planetary Sciences* **43**, 405–429, doi:10.1146/annurev-earth-060614-105310 (2015).

271 Maslin, M. A. *et al.* East African climate pulses and early human evolution. *Quat. Sci. Rev.* **101**, 1–17, doi:10.1016/j.quascirev.2014.06.012 (2014).

272 Potts, R. Variability selection in hominid evolution. *Evol. Anthropol.* **7**, 81–96, doi:10.1002/(sici)1520-6505(1998)7:3<81::aid-evan3>3.0.co;2-a (1998).

273 Potts, R. Environmental hypotheses of hominin evolution. *Yearbook of Physical Anthropology* **41**, 93–136 (1998).

274 Sterelny, K. Language, gesture, skill: the co-evolutionary foundations of language. *Philos. Trans. R. Soc. B-Biol. Sci.* **367**, 2141–2151, doi:10.1098/rstb.2012.0116 (2012).

275 Sterelny, K. Social intelligence, human intelligence and niche construction. *Philos. Trans. R. Soc. B-Biol. Sci.* **362**, 719–730, doi:10.1098/rstb.2006.2006 (2007).

276 Sterelny, K. From hominins to humans: how sapiens became behaviourally modern. *Philos. Trans. R. Soc. B-Biol. Sci.* **366**, 809–822, doi:10.1098/rstb.2010.0301 (2011).

277 Whiten, A. & Erdal, D. The human socio-cognitive niche and its evolutionary origins. *Philos. Trans. R. Soc. B-Biol. Sci.* **367**, 2119–2129, doi:10.1098/rstb.2012.0114 (2012).

278 Marwick, B. Pleistocene exchange networks as evidence for the evolution of language. *Cambridge Archaeological Journal* **13**, 67–81, doi:10.1017/s0959774303000040 (2003).

279 Bulut, S. Intelligence development of socio-economically disadvantaged pre-school children. *Anales De Psicologia* **29**, 855–864, doi:10.6018/analesps.29.3.168101 (2013).

280 Cattell, R. B. *Abilities: Their structure, growth, and action* (Houghton Mifflin, 1971).

281 Deary, I. J., Strand, S., Smith, P. & Fernandes, C. Intelligence and educational achievement. *Intelligence* **35**, 13–21, doi:10.1016/j.intell.2006.02.001 (2007).

282 Rohde, T. E. & Thompson, L. A. Predicting academic achievement with cognitive ability. *Intelligence* **35**, 83–92, doi:10.1016/j.intell.2006.05.004 (2007).

283 Bouchard, T. J. Genes, Evolution and intelligence. *Behavior Genetics* **44**, 549–577, doi:10.1007/s10519-014-9646-x (2014).

284 Ash, J. & Gallup, G. G. Paleoclimatic variation and brain expansion during human evolution. *Hum. Nat.-Interdiscip. Biosoc. Perspect.* **18**, 109–124, doi:10.1007/s12110-007-9015-z (2007).

285 Shultz, S., Nelson, E. & Dunbar, R. I. M. Hominin cognitive evolution: identifying patterns and processes in the fossil and archaeological record. *Philos. Trans. R. Soc. B-Biol. Sci.* **367**, 2130–2140, doi:10.1098/rstb.2012.0115 (2012).

286 Mitani, J. C. Demographic influences on the behavior of chimpanzees. *Primates* **47**, 6–13, doi:10.1007/s10329-005-0139-7 (2006).

287 Boesch, C. Cooperative hunting in wild chimpanzees. *Anim. Behav.* **48**, 653–667, doi:10.1006/anbe.1994.1285 (1994).

288 Jaeggi, A. V., Burkart, J. M. & Van Schaik, C. P. On the psychology of cooperation in humans and other primates: combining the natural history and experimental evidence of prosociality. *Philos. Trans. R. Soc. B-Biol. Sci.* **365**, 2723–2735, doi:10.1098/rstb.2010.0118 (2010).

289 Ueno, A. & Matsuzawa, T. Food transfer between chimpanzee mothers and their infants. *Primates* **45**, 231–239, doi:10.1007/s10329-004-0085-9 (2004).

290 Coall, D. A. & Hertwig, R. Grandparental investment: past, present, and future. *Behav. Brain Sci.* **33**, 1, doi:10.1017/s0140525x09991105 (2010).

291 Kramer, K. L. in *Annual Review of Anthropology*, Vol. 39 (eds D. Brenneis & P. T. Ellison), 417–436 (Annual Reviews, 2010).

292 Sear, R. & Mace, R. Who keeps children alive? A review of the effects of kin on child survival. *Evol. Hum. Behav.* **29**, 1–18, doi:10.1016/j.evolhumbehav.2007.10.001 (2008).

293 Gurven, M. & Hill, K. Why do men hunt? A reevaluation of "man the hunter" and the sexual division of labor. *Curr. Anthropol.* **50**, 51–74, doi:10.1086/595620 (2009).

294 Marlowe, F. W. Hunter-gatherers and human evolution. *Evol. Anthropol.* **14**, 54–67, doi:10.1002/evan.20046 (2005).

295 Kaplan, H. S., Hooper, P. L. & Gurven, M. The evolutionary and ecological roots of human social organization. *Philos. Trans. R. Soc. B-Biol. Sci.* **364**, 3289–3299, doi:10.1098/rstb.2009.0115 (2009).

296 Hill, K. & Hurtado, A. M. Cooperative breeding in South American hunter-gatherers. *Proc. R. Soc. B-Biol. Sci.* **276**, 3863–3870, doi:10.1098/rspb.2009.1061 (2009).

297 Burkart, J. M. & Finkenwirth, C. Marmosets as model species in neuroscience and evolutionary anthropology. *Neuroscience Research* **93**, 8–19, doi:10.1016/j.neures.2014.09.003 (2015).

298 Digby, L. J., Ferrari, S. F. & Saltzman, W. in *Primates in perspective* (eds C. J. Campbell, A. Fuentes & K. C. Mackinnon), 85–105 (Oxford University Press, 2007).

299 Burkart, J. M., Fehr, E., Efferson, C. & van Schaik, C. P. Other-regarding preferences in a non-human primate: common marmosets provision food altruistically. *Proc. Natl. Acad. Sci. U.S.A.* **104**, 19762–19766, doi:10.1073/pnas.0710310104 (2007).

300 Clutton-Brock, T. Behavioral ecology: breeding together: kin selection and mutualism in cooperative vertebrates. *Science* **296**, 69–72, doi:10.1126/science.296.5565.69 (2002).

301 Faulkes, C. G., Arruda, M. F. & Monteiro da Cruz, M. A. O. *Genetic structure within and among populations of the common marmoset, Callithrix jacchus: Implications for cooperative breeding* (Springer, 2009).

302 Fite, J. E. *et al.* Nighttime wakefulness associated with infant rearing in Callithrix kuhlii. *International Journal of Primatology* **24**, 1267–1280, doi:10.1023/B:IJOP.0000005992.72026.e6 (2003).

303 Fite, J. E. *et al.* Opportunistic mothers: female marmosets (Callithrix kuhlii) reduce their investment in offspring when they have to, and when they can. *J. Hum. Evol.* **49**, 122–142, doi:10.1016/j.jhevol.2005.04.003 (2005).

304 Martins, E. M. G. & Burkart, J. M. Common marmosets preferentially share difficult to obtain food items. *Folia Primatol.* **84**, 281–282 (2013).

305 Voelkl, B., Schrauf, C. & Huber, L. Social contact influences the response of infant marmosets towards novel food. *Anim. Behav.* **72**, 365–372, doi:10.1016/j.anbehav.2005.10.013 (2006).

306 Brown, G. R., Almond, R. E. A. & Van Bergen, Y. Begging, stealing, and offering: food transfer in nonhuman primates. *Advances in the Study of Behavior* **34**, 265–295, doi:10.1016/s0065-3454(04)34007-6 (2004).

307 Joyce, S. M. & Snowdon, C. T. Developmental changes in food transfers in cotton-top tamarins (Saguinus oedipus). *American Journal of Primatology* **69**, 955–965, doi:10.1002/ajp.20393 (2007).

308 Snowdon, C. T. Social processes in communication and cognition in callitrichid monkeys: a review. *Anim. Cogn.* **4**, 247–257, doi:10.1007/s100710100094 (2001).

309 Burkart, J. M. *et al.* The evolutionary origin of human hyper-cooperation. *Nat. Commun.* **5**, doi:10.1038/ncomms5747 (2014).

310 Curley, J. P. & Keverne, E. B. Genes, brains and mammalian social bonds. *Trends Ecol. Evol.* **20**, 561–567, doi:10.1016/j.tree.2005.05.018 (2005).

311 Broad, K. D., Curley, J. P. & Keverne, E. B. Mother-infant bonding and the evolution of mammalian social relationships. *Philos. Trans. R. Soc. B-Biol. Sci.* **361**, 2199–2214, doi:10.1098/rstb.2006.1940 (2006).

312 Crockford, C. *et al.* Urinary oxytocin and social bonding in related and unrelated wild chimpanzees. *Proceedings of the Royal Society of London B: Biological Sciences* **280**, doi:10.1098/rspb.2012.2765 (2013).

313 Finkenwirth, C., van Schaik, C. & Burkart, J. Relationships in common marmoset families: oxytocin synchronicity is linked to dyadic bond strength. *Folia Primatol.* **84**, 273 (2013).

314 Baumgartner, T., Heinrichs, M., Vonlanthen, A., Fischbacher, U. & Fehr, E. Oxytocin shapes the neural circuitry of trust and trust adaptation in humans. *Neuron* **58**, 639–650, doi:10.1016/j.neuron.2008.04.009 (2008).

315 Kosfeld, M., Heinrichs, M., Zak, P. J., Fischbacher, U. & Fehr, E. Oxytocin increases trust in humans. *Nature* **435**, 673–676, doi:10.1038/nature03701 (2005).

316 Zak, P. J., Stanton, A. A. & Ahmadi, S. Oxytocin increases generosity in humans. *PLOS One* **2**, 5, doi:10.1371/journal.pone.0001128 (2007).

317 Saito, A. & Nakamura, K. Oxytocin changes primate paternal tolerance to offspring in food transfer. *J. Comp. Physiol. A Neuroethol. Sens. Neural Behav. Physiol.* **197**, 329–337, doi:10.1007/s00359-010-0617-2 (2011).

318 Chang, S. W. C., Barter, J. W., Ebitz, R. B., Watson, K. K. & Platt, M. L. Inhaled oxytocin amplifies both vicarious reinforcement and self reinforcement in rhesus macaques (Macaca mulatta). *Proc. Natl. Acad. Sci. U.S.A.* **109**, 959–964, doi:10.1073/pnas.1114621109 (2012).

319 Ebitz, R. B., Watson, K. K. & Platt, M. L. Oxytocin blunts social vigilance in the rhesus macaque. *Proc. Natl. Acad. Sci. U.S.A.* **110**, 11630–11635, doi:10.1073/pnas.1305230110 (2013).

320 Mohiyeddini, C., Opacka-Juffry, J. & Gross, J. J. Emotional suppression explains the link between early life stress and plasma oxytocin. *Anxiety Stress Coping* **27**, 466–475, doi:10.1080/10615806.2014.887696 (2014).

321 De Dreu, C. K. W., Greer, L. L., Van Kleef, G. A., Shalvi, S. & Handgraaf, M. J. J. Oxytocin promotes human ethnocentrism. *Proc. Natl. Acad. Sci. U.S.A.* **108**, 1262–1266, doi:10.1073/pnas.1015316108 (2011).

322 Declerck, C. H., Boone, C. & Kiyonari, T. Oxytocin and cooperation under conditions of uncertainty: the modulating role of incentives and social information. *Horm. Behav.* **57**, 368–374, doi:10.1016/j.yhbeh.2010.01.006 (2010).

323 Declerck, C. H., Boone, C. & Kiyonari, T. The effect of oxytocin on cooperation in a prisoner's dilemma depends on the social context and a person's social value orientation. *Social Cognitive and Affective Neuroscience* **9**, 802–809, doi:10.1093/scan/nst040 (2014).

324 Burkart, J. M. & van Schaik, C. Group service in macaques (Macaca fuscata), capuchins (Cebus apella) and marmosets (Callithrix jacchus): a comparative approach to identifying proactive prosocial motivations. *J. Comp. Psychol.* **127**, 212–225, doi:10.1037/a0026392 (2013).

325 Koenig, A. Random scan, sentinels or sentinel system? A study in captive common marmosets (Callithrix jacchus). *Current Primatology* **2**, 69–76 (1994).

326 Goldizen, A. W. in *Primate societies* (eds B. B. Smuts, D. L. Cheney & R. M. Seyfarth), 34–43 (1987).

327 Willems, E. P., Hellriegel, B. & van Schaik, C. P. The collective action problem in primate territory economics. *Proc. R. Soc. B-Biol. Sci.* **280**, 7, doi:10.1098/rspb.2013.0081 (2013).

328 Garber, P. A. One for all and breeding for one: cooperation and competition as a tamarin reproductive strategy. *Evolutionary Anthropology: Issues, News, and Reviews* **5**, 187–199, doi:10.1002/(SICI)1520-6505(1997)5:6<187::AID-EVAN1>3.0.CO;2-A (1997).

329 Rapaport, L. G. & Brown, G. R. Social influences on foraging behavior in young nonhuman primates: learning what, where, and how to eat. *Evol. Anthropol.* **17**, 189–201, doi:10.1002/evan.20180 (2008).

330 Rapaport, L. G. Progressive parenting behavior in wild golden lion tamarins. *Behavioral Ecology* **22**, 745–754, doi:10.1093/beheco/arr055 (2011).

331 Humle, T. & Snowdon, C. T. Socially biased learning in the acquisition of a complex foraging task in juvenile cottontop tamarins, Saguinus oedipus. *Anim. Behav.* **75**, 267–277, doi:10.1016/j.anbehav.2007.05.021 (2008).

332 Thornton, A. & McAuliffe, K. Cognitive consequences of cooperative breeding? A critical appraisal. *Journal of Zoology* **295**, 12–22, doi:10.1111/jzo.12198 (2015).

333 Dillis, C., Humle, T. & Snowdon, C. T. Socially biased learning among adult cottontop tamarins (Saguinus oedipus). *American Journal of Primatology* **72**, 287–295, doi:10.1002/ajp.20778 (2010).

334 Moll, H. & Tomasello, M. Cooperation and human cognition: the Vygotskian intelligence hypothesis. *Philos. Trans. R. Soc. B-Biol. Sci.* **362**, 639–648, doi:10.1098/rstb.2006.2000 (2007).

335 Lefebvre, L. & Giraldeau, L. A. in *Social learning in animals: The roots of culture* (eds C. M. Heyes Jr & B. G. Galef Jr), 107–128 (Academic Press, 1996).

336 Boogert, N. J., Giraldeau, L. A. & Lefebvre, L. Song complexity correlates with learning ability in zebra finch males. *Anim. Behav.* **76**, 1735–1741, doi:10.1016/j.anbehav.2008.08.009 (2008).

337 Bouchard, J., Goodyer, W. & Lefebvre, L. Social learning and innovation are positively correlated in pigeons (Columba livia). *Anim. Cogn.* **10**, 259–266, doi:10.1007/s10071-006-0064-1 (2007).

338 Wilkinson, A., Kuenstner, K., Mueller, J. & Huber, L. Social learning in a non-social reptile (Geochelone carbonaria). *Biol. Lett.* **6**, 614–616, doi:10.1098/rsbl.2010.0092 (2010).

339 Yuill, N., Hinske, S., Williams, S. E. & Leith, G. How getting noticed helps getting on: successful attention capture doubles children's cooperative play. *Frontiers in Psychology* **5**, doi:10.3389/fpsyg.2014.00418 (2014).

340 Jack, R. E., Blais, C., Scheepers, C., Schyns, P. G. & Caldara, R. Cultural confusions show that facial expressions are not universal. *Curr. Biol.* **19**, 1543–1548, doi:10.1016/j.cub.2009.07.051 (2009).

341 Deák, G. O. & Triesch, J. in *Diversity of cognition* (eds K. Fujita & S. Itakura), 331–363 (University of Kyoto Press, 2006).

342 Oberwelland, E. *et al.* Look into my eyes: investigating joint attention using interactive eye-tracking and fMRI in a developmental sample. *Neuroimage* **130**, 248–260, doi:10.1016/j.neuroimage.2016.02.026 (2016).

343 Triesch, J., Teuscher, C., Deak, G. O. & Carlson, E. Gaze following: why (not) learn it? *Dev. Sci.* **9**, 125–147, doi:10.1111/j.1467-7687.2006.00470.x (2006).

344 Adapted from Stout, D. & Chaminade, T. The evolutionary neuroscience of tool making. *Neuropsychologia* **14**, 45, 1091–1100 (2007).

345 Delagnes, A. & Roche, H. Late Pliocene hominid knapping skills: the case of Lokalalei 2C, West Turkana, Kenya. *J. Hum. Evol.* **48**, 435–472, doi:dx.doi.org/10.1016/j.jhevol.2004.12.005 (2005).

346 Semaw, S. *et al.* 2.5-million-year-old stone tools from Gona, Ethiopia. *Nature* **385**, 333–336, doi:10.1038/385333a0 (1997).

347 Leakey, M. D. *Olduvai Gorge volume 3: Excavations in Beds I and II, 1960–1963* (Cambridge University Press, 1971).

348 Isaac, G. L. & Isaac, B. *Koobi fora research project* (Clarendon Press, 1997).

349 Braun, D. R. & Hovers, E. in *Interdisciplinary approaches to the Oldowan vertebrate paleobiology and paleoanthropology* (eds E. Hovers & D. R. Braun), 1–14 (Springer, 2009).

350 Sahnouni, M. in *The Oldowan: Case studies into the earliest Stone Age* (eds N. Toth & K. Schick), 77–111 (Stone Age Institute Press, 2006).

351 Kuman, K. in *Breathing life into fossils: Taphonomic studies in honor of C. K. (Bob) Brain* (eds T. R. Schick, K. Pickering & N. Toth), 181–198 (Stone Age Institute Press, 2007).

352 Stout, D., Semaw, S., Rogers, M. J. & Cauche, D. Technological variation in the earliest Oldowan from Gona, Afar, Ethiopia. *J. Hum. Evol.* **58**, 474–491, doi:dx.doi.org/10.1016/j.jhevol.2010.02.005 (2010).

353 Adapted from Stout, D. *et al.*, Neural correlates of Early Stone Age toolmaking: technology, language and cognition in human evolution. *Philos. Trans. R. Soc. Lond. B. Biol. Sci.* **363**, 1499, 1939–1949 (2008).

354 Lieberman, P. Language did not spring forth 100,000 years ago. *PLoS Biol.* **13**, 4, doi:10.1371/journal.pbio.1002064 (2015).

355 Morgan, T. J. H. *et al.* Experimental evidence for the co-evolution of hominin tool-making teaching and language. *Nature Communications* **6**, 8, doi:10.1038/ncomms7029 (2015).

356 Issar, A. S. Climate change as a draw bridge between Africa and the Middle East. *Glob. Planet. Change* **72**, 451–454, doi:10.1016/j.gloplacha.2010.01.018 (2010).

357 Zhu, R. X. *et al.* Early evidence of the genus Homo in East Asia. *J. Hum. Evol.* **55**, 1075–1085, doi:dx.doi.org/10.1016/j.jhevol.2008.08.005 (2008).

358 Stringer, C. The chronological and evolutionary position of the Broken Hill cranium. *American Journal of Physical Anthropology* **144**, 287 (2011).

359 Clark, J. D. *et al.* African Homo-erectus: old radiometric ages and young Oldowan assemblages in the middle-Awash valley, Ethiopia. *Science* **264**, 1907–1910, doi:10.1126/science.8009220 (1994).

360 Rightmire, G. P. The human cranium from Bodo, Ethiopia: evidence for speciation in the Middle Pleistocene? *J. Hum. Evol.* **31**, 21–39 (1996).

361 Stringer, C. The status of Homo heidelbergensis (Schoetensack 1908). *Evol. Anthropol.* **21**, 101–107, doi:10.1002/evan.21311 (2012).

362 White, T. D. *et al.* Pleistocene Homo sapiens from Middle Awash, Ethiopia. *Nature* **423**, 742–747, doi:10.1038/nature01669 (2003).

363 McDougall, I., Brown, F. H. & Fleagle, J. G. Stratigraphic placement and age of modern humans from Kibish, Ethiopia. *Nature* **433**, 733–736, doi:10.1038/nature03258 (2005).

364 Wood, B. & Leakey, M. The Omo-Turkana basin fossil Hominins and their contribution to our understanding of human evolution in Africa. *Evol. Anthropol.* **20**, 264–292, doi:10.1002/evan.20335 (2011).

365 Henn, B. M., Cavalli-Sforza, L. L. & Feldman, M. W. The great human expansion. *Proc. Natl. Acad. Sci. U.S.A.* **109**, 17758–17764, doi:10.1073/pnas.1212380109 (2012).

366 Klein, R. G. Whither the Neanderthals? *Science* **299**, 1525–1527, doi:10.1126/science.1082025 (2003).

367 Green, R. E. *et al.* A draft sequence of the Neandertal genome. *Science* **328**, 710–722, doi:10.1126/science.1188021 (2010).

368 Reich, D. *et al.* Genetic history of an archaic hominin group from Denisova Cave in Siberia. *Nature* **468**, 1053–1060, doi:10.1038/nature09710 (2010).

369 Weaver, T. D., Roseman, C. C. & Stringer, C. B. Close correspondence between quantitative- and molecular-genetic divergence times for Neandertals and modern humans. *Proc. Natl. Acad. Sci. U.S.A.* **105**, 4645–4649, doi:10.1073/pnas.0709079105 (2008).

370 Krings, M. *et al.* Neandertal DNA sequences and the origin of modern humans. *Cell* **90**, 19–30, doi:10.1016/s0092-8674(00)80310-4 (1997).

371 Serre, D. *et al.* No evidence of neandertal mtDNA contribution to early modern humans. *PLoS Biol.* **2**, 313–317, doi:10.1371/journal.pbio.0020057 (2004).

372 Green, R. E. *et al.* Analysis of one million base pairs of Neanderthal DNA. *Nature* **444**, 330–336, doi:10.1038/nature05336 (2006).

373 Green, R. E. *et al.* A complete neandertal mitochondrial genome sequence determined by high-throughput Sequencing. *Cell* **134**, 416–426, doi:10.1016/j.cell.2008.06.021 (2008).

374 Noonan, J. P. *et al.* Sequencing and analysis of Neanderthal genomic DNA. *Science* **314**, 1113–1118, doi:10.1126/science.1131412 (2006).

375 Gell-Mann, M. & Ruhlen, M. The origin and evolution of word order. *Proc. Natl. Acad. Sci. U.S.A.* **108**, 17290–17295, doi:10.1073/pnas.1113716108 (2011).

376 Atkinson, Q. D. Phonemic diversity supports a serial founder effect model of language expansion from Africa. *Science* **332**, 346–349, doi:10.1126/science.1199295 (2011).

377 Creanza, N. *et al.* A comparison of worldwide phonemic and genetic variation in human populations. *Proc. Natl. Acad. Sci. U.S.A.* **112**, 1265–1272, doi:10.1073/pnas.1424033112 (2015).

378 Goldin-Meadow, S., Goodrich, W., Sauer, E. & Iverson, J. Young children use their hands to tell their mothers what to say. *Dev. Sci.* **10**, 778–785, doi:10.1111/j.1467-7687.2007.00636.x (2007).

379 Iverson, J. M. & Goldin-Meadow, S. Gesture paves the way for language development. *Psychological Science* **16**, 367–371, doi:10.1111/j.0956-7976.2005.01542.x (2005).

380 Novack, M. & Goldin-Meadow, S. Learning from gesture: how our hands change our minds. *Educational Psychology Review* **27**, 405–412, doi:10.1007/s10648-015-9325-3 (2015).

381 Bass, A. H. & Chagnaud, B. P. Shared developmental and evolutionary origins for neural basis of vocal-acoustic and pectoral-gestural signaling. *Proc. Natl. Acad. Sci. U.S.A.* **109**, 10677–10684, doi:10.1073/pnas.1201886109 (2012).

382 Iverson, J. M. & Thelen, E. Hand, mouth and brain: the dynamic emergence of speech and gesture. *Journal of Consciousness Studies* **6**, 19–40 (1999).

383 Kroliczak, G., Piper, B. J. & Frey, S. H. Atypical lateralization of language predicts cerebral asymmetries in parietal gesture representations. *Neuropsychologia* **49**, 1698–1702, doi:10.1016/j.neuropsychologia.2011.02.044 (2011).

384 Vingerhoets, G. *et al.* Praxis and language are linked: evidence from co-lateralization in individuals, with atypical language dominance. *Cortex* **49**, 172–183, doi:10.1016/j.cortex.2011.11.003 (2013).

385 Goldstone, R. L. & Son, J. Y. The transfer of scientific principles using concrete and idealized simulations. *J. Learn. Sci.* **14**, 69–110, doi:10.1207/s15327809jls1401_4 (2005).

386 Moreno, R., Ozogul, G. & Reisslein, M. Teaching with concrete and abstract visual representations: effects on students' problem solving, problem representations, and learning perceptions. *Journal of Educational Psychology* **103**, 32–47, doi:10.1037/a0021995 (2011).

387 McNeil, N. M. & Fyfe, E. R. "Concreteness fading" promotes transfer of mathematical knowledge. *Learning and Instruction* **22**, 440–448, doi:10.1016/j.learninstruc.2012.05.001 (2012).

388 Flaugnacco, E. *et al.* Music training increases phonological awareness and reading skills in developmental dyslexia: a randomized control trial. *PLOS One* **10**, 17, doi:10.1371/journal.pone.0138715 (2015).

389 Leong, V. & Goswami, U. Acoustic-emergent phonology in the amplitude envelope of child-directed speech. *PLOS One* **10**, 37, doi:10.1371/journal.pone.0144411 (2015).

390 Thomson, J. M., Leong, V. & Goswami, U. Auditory processing interventions and developmental dyslexia: a comparison of phonemic and rhythmic approaches. *Reading and Writing* **26**, 139–161, doi:10.1007/s11145-012-9359-6 (2013).

391 Bhide, A., Power, A. & Goswami, U. A rhythmic musical intervention for poor readers: a comparison of efficacy with a letter-based intervention. *Mind, Brain, and Education* **7**, 113–123, doi:10.1111/mbe.12016 (2013).

392 Larsson, M. Tool-use-associated sound in the evolution of language. *Anim. Cogn.* **18**, 993–1005, doi:10.1007/s10071-015-0885-x (2015).

393 Nowicki, S. & Searcy, W. A. The evolution of vocal learning. *Curr. Opin. Neurobiol.* **28**, 48–53, doi:dx.doi.org/10.1016/j.conb.2014.06.007 (2014).

394 Darwin, C. R. *The descent of man and selection in relation to sex* (John Murray, 1871).

395 Fitch, W. T. *The evolution of language* (Cambridge University Press, 2010).

396 Ackermann, H., Hage, S. R. & Ziegler, W. Brain mechanisms of acoustic communication in humans and nonhuman primates: an evolutionary perspective. *Behav. Brain Sci.* **37**, 71, doi:10.1017/s0140525x13003099 (2014).

397 Enard, W. *et al.* A humanized version of Foxp2 affects cortico-basal ganglia circuits in mice. *Cell* **137**, 961–971, doi:10.1016/j.cell.2009.03.041 (2009).

398 Lieberman, P. The evolution of human speech: its anatomical and neural bases. *Curr. Anthropol.* **48**, 39–66, doi:10.1086/509092 (2007).

399 Maricic, T. *et al.* A recent evolutionary change affects a regulatory element in the human FOXP2 gene. *Molecular Biology and Evolution* **30**, 844–852, doi:10.1093/molbev/mss271 (2013).

400 Dediu, D. & Levinson, S. C. On the antiquity of language: the reinterpretation of Neandertal linguistic capacities and its consequences. *Frontiers in Psychology* **4**, 17, doi:10.3389/fpsyg.2013.00397 (2013).

401 Johansson, S. in *Annual Review of Linguistics*, Vol. 1 (eds M. Liberman & B. H. Partee), 311–332 (Annual Reviews, 2015).

402 Fisher, S. E. Dissection of molecular mechanisms underlying speech and language disorders. *Appl. Psycholinguist.* **26**, 111–128, doi:10.1017/s014271640 5050095 (2005).

403 Coward, F. & Gamble, C. Big brains, small worlds: material culture and the evolution of the mind. *Philos. Trans. R. Soc. B-Biol. Sci.* **363**, 1969–1979, doi:10.1098/rstb.2008.0004 (2008).

404 Ingold, T. *The perception of the environment: Essays in livelihood, dwelling and skill* (Routledge, 2000).

405 Tomblin, J. B. *et al.* Prevalence of specific language impairment in kindergarten children. *J. Speech Lang. Hear. Res.* **40**, 1245–1260 (1997).

406 Arcos-Burgos, M. & Acosta, M. T. Tuning major gene variants conditioning human behavior: the anachronism of ADHD. *Curr. Opin. Genet. Dev.* **17**, 234–238, doi:dx.doi.org/10.1016/j.gde.2007.04.011 (2007).

407 Bishop, D. V. M. in *Year in Cognitive Neuroscience*, Vol. 1156, *Annals of the New York Academy of Sciences* (eds M. B. Miller & A. Kingstone), 1–18 (2009).

408 Bishop, D. V. M. The interface between genetics and psychology: lessons from developmental dyslexia. *Proc. R. Soc. B-Biol. Sci.* **282**, 8, doi:10.1098/rspb.2014.3139 (2015).

409 Wright, A., Charlesworth, B., Rudan, I., Carothers, A. & Campbell, H. A polygenic basis for late-onset disease. *Trends in Genetics* **19**, 97–106, doi:dx.doi.org/10.1016/S0168-9525(02)00033-1 (2003).

410 Plomin, R., Kovas, Y. & Haworth, C. M. A. Generalist genes: genetic links between brain, mind, and education. *Mind, Brain, and Education* **1**, 11–19 (2007).

411 Plomin, R. & Kovas, Y. Generalist genes and learning disabilities. *Psychological Bulletin* **131**, 592–617, doi:10.1037/0033-2909.131.4.592 (2005).

412 Schilbach, L. *et al.* Minds made for sharing: initiating joint attention recruits reward-related neurocircuitry. *Journal of Cognitive Neuroscience* **22**, 2702–2715, doi:10.1162/jocn.2009.21401 (2010).

413 Roebroeks, W. *et al.* Use of red ochre by early Neandertals. *Proc. Natl. Acad. Sci. U.S.A.*, doi:10.1073/pnas.1112261109 (2012).

414 Morin, E. & Laroulandie, V. Presumed symbolic use of diurnal raptors by Neanderthals. *PLOS One* **7**, e32856, doi:10.1371/journal.pone.0032856 (2012).

415 Finlayson, C. *et al.* Birds of a feather: Neanderthal exploitation of raptors and corvids. *PLOS One* **7**, e45927, doi:10.1371/journal.pone.0045927 (2012).

416 Lieberman, P. Vocal tract anatomy and the neural bases of talking. *J. Phon.* **40**, 608–622, doi:10.1016/j.wocn.2012.04.001 (2012).

417 d'Errico, F. & Stringer, C. B. Evolution, revolution or saltation scenario for the emergence of modern cultures? *Philos. Trans. R. Soc. B-Biol. Sci.* **366**, 1060–1069, doi:10.1098/rstb.2010.0340 (2011).

418 Mellars, P. Why did modern human populations disperse from Africa ca. 60,000 years ago? A new model. *Proc. Natl. Acad. Sci. U.S.A.* **103**, 13560–13560, doi:10.1073/pnas.0605126103 (2006).

419 Boyd, R., Richerson, P. J. & Henrich, J. The cultural niche: why social learning is essential for human adaptation. *Proc. Natl. Acad. Sci. U.S.A.* **108**, 10918–10925, doi:10.1073/pnas.1100290108 (2011).

420 Kolodny, O., Creanza, N. & Feldman, M. W. Evolution in leaps: the punctuated accumulation and loss of cultural innovations. *Proc. Natl. Acad. Sci. U.S.A.* **112**, E6762-E6769, doi:10.1073/pnas.1520492112 (2015).

421 Henrich, J. Demography and cultural evolution: how adaptive cultural processes can produce maladaptive losses: the Tasmanian case. *American Antiquity* **69**, 197–214, doi:10.2307/4128416 (2004).

422 Kline, M. A. & Boyd, R. Population size predicts technological complexity in Oceania. *Proc. R. Soc. B-Biol. Sci.* **277**, 2559–2564, doi:10.1098/rspb.2010.0452 (2010).

423 Rasmussen, K. *The people of the polar north* (Kegan Paul, 1908).

424 Mary-Rousselière, G. *Qitdlarssuaq: The story of a polar migration* (Wuerz Publishing, 1996).

425 Tennie, C., Call, J. & Tomasello, M. Ratcheting up the ratchet: on the evolution of cumulative culture. *Philos. Trans. R. Soc. B-Biol. Sci.* **364**, 2405–2415, doi:10.1098/rstb.2009.0052 (2009).

426 Derex, M., Beugin, M. P., Godelle, B. & Raymond, M. Experimental evidence for the influence of group size on cultural complexity. *Nature* **503**, 389, doi:10.1038/nature12774 (2013).

427 Derex, M. & Boyd, R. The foundations of the human cultural niche. *Nature Communications* **6**, 7, doi:10.1038/ncomms9398 (2015).

428 Fink, A. *et al.* Enhancing creativity by means of cognitive stimulation: evidence from an fMRI study. *Neuroimage* **52**, 1687–1695, doi:10.1016/j.neuroimage.2010.05.072 (2010).

429 Shoshani, J., Kupsky, W. J. & Marchant, G. H. Elephant brain: part 1: gross morphology, functions, comparative anatomy, and evolution. *Brain Res. Bull.* **70**, 124–157, doi:10.1016/j.brainresbull.2006.03.016 (2006).

430 Marino, L. A comparison of encephalization between odontocete cetaceans and anthropoid primates. *Brain Behav. Evol.* **51**, 230–238, doi:10.1159/000006540 (1998).

431 Kaufmann, L. *et al.* Developmental dyscalculia: compensatory mechanisms in left intraparietal regions in response to nonsymbolic magnitudes. *Behavioral and Brain Functions* **5**, 35, doi:10.1186/1744-9081-5-35 (2009).

432 Stephan, H., Frahm, H. & Baron, G. New and revised data on volumes of brain structures in insectivores and primates. *Folia Primatol.* **35**, 1–29, doi:10.1159/000155963 (1981).

433 Hofman, M. A. Size and shape of the cerebral-cortex in mammals. 1. The cortical surface. *Brain Behav. Evol.* **27**, 28–40, doi:10.1159/000118718 (1985).

434 Kucian, K. *et al.* Impaired neural networks for approximate calculation in dyscalculic children: a functional MRI study. *Behavioral and Brain Functions: BBF* **2**, 31–31, doi:10.1186/1744-9081-2-31 (2006).

435 Mussolin, C. *et al.* Neural correlates of symbolic number comparison in developmental dyscalculia. *Journal of Cognitive Neuroscience* **22**, 860–874, doi:10.1162/jocn.2009.21237 (2010).

436 Price, G. R., Holloway, I., Raesaenen, P., Vesterinen, M. & Ansari, D. Impaired parietal magnitude processing in developmental dyscalculia. *Curr. Biol.* **17**, R1042-R1043, doi:10.1016/j.cub.2007.10.013 (2007).

437 Rotzer, S. *et al.* Optimized voxel-based morphometry in children with developmental dyscalculia. *Neuroimage* **39**, 417–422, doi:10.1016/j.neuroimage.2007.08.045 (2008).

438 Soltesz, F., Szucs, D. & Szucs, L. Relationships between magnitude representation, counting and memory in 4- to 7-year-old children: a developmental study. *Behavioral and Brain Functions* **6**, doi:10.1186/1744-9081-6-13 (2010).

439 Herculano-Houzel, S. *et al.* Updated neuronal scaling rules for the brains of glires (Rodents/Lagomorphs). *Brain Behav. Evol.* **78**, 302–314, doi:10.1159/000330825 (2011).

440 Sarko, D. K., Catania, K. C., Leitch, D. B., Kaas, J. H. & Herculano-Houzel, S. Cellular scaling rules of insectivore brains. *Front. Neuroanat.* **3**, doi:810.3389/neuro.05.008.2009 (2009).

441 Herculano-Houzel, S. The remarkable, yet not extraordinary, human brain as a scaled-up primate brain and its associated cost. *Proc. Natl. Acad. Sci. U.S.A.* **109**, 10661–10668, doi:10.1073/pnas.1201895109 (2012).

442 Holloway, R. L., Sherwood, C. C., Hof, P. R. & Rilling, J. K. in *The new encyclopedia of neuroscience* (Springer, 2009).

443 Herculano-Houzel, S. & Kaas, J. H. Gorilla and orangutan brains conform to the primate cellular scaling rules: implications for human evolution. *Brain Behav. Evol.* **77**, 33–44, doi:10.1159/000322729 (2011).

444 Herculano-Houzel, S. Not all brains are made the same: new views on brain scaling in evolution. *Brain Behav. Evol.* **78**, 22–36, doi:10.1159/000327318 (2011).

445 Anderson, J. R., Awazu, S. & Fujita, K. Can squirrel monkeys (Saimiri sciureus) learn self-control? A study using food array selection tests and reverse-reward contingency. *J. Exp. Psychol.-Anim. Behav. Process.* **26**, 87–97, doi:10.1037/0097-7403.26.1.87 (2000).

446 Beran, M. J., McIntyre, J. M., Garland, A. & Evans, T. A. What counts for 'counting'? Chimpanzees, Pan troglodytes, respond appropriately to relevant and irrelevant information in a quantity judgment task. *Anim. Behav.* **85**, 987–993, doi:10.1016/j.anbehav.2013.02.022 (2013).

447 Beran, M. J., Perdue, B. M., Parrish, A. E. & Evans, T. A. Do social conditions affect capuchin monkeys' (Cebus apella) choices in a quantity judgment task? *Frontiers in Psychology* **3**, doi:10.3389/fpsyg.2012.00492 (2012).

448 Bonanni, R., Natoli, E., Cafazzo, S. & Valsecchi, P. Free-ranging dogs assess the quantity of opponents in intergroup conflicts. *Anim. Cogn.* **14**, 103–115, doi:10.1007/s10071-010-0348-3 (2011).

449 Garland, A., Low, J. & Burns, K. C. Large quantity discrimination by North Island robins (Petroica longipes). *Anim. Cogn.* **15**, 1129–1140, doi:10.1007/s10071-012-0537-3 (2012).

450 Hunt, S., Low, J. & Burns, K. C. Adaptive numerical competency in a food-hoarding songbird. *Proc. R. Soc. B-Biol. Sci.* **275**, 2373–2379, doi:10.1098/rspb.2008.0702 (2008).

451 Agrillo, C., Miletto Petrazzini, M. & Bisazza, A. Numerical acuity of fish is improved in the presence of moving targets, but only in the subitizing range. *Anim. Cogn.* **17**, 307–316, doi:10.1007/s10071-013-0663-6 (2014).

452 Bisazza, A., Agrillo, C. & Lucon-Xiccato, T. Extensive training extends numerical abilities of guppies. *Anim. Cogn.* **17**, 1413–1419, doi:10.1007/s10071-014-0759-7 (2014).

453 Scholl, B. J. & Pylyshyn, Z. W. Tracking multiple items through occlusion: Clues to visual objecthood. *Cognitive Psychology* **38**, 259–290, doi:10.1006/cogp.1998.0698 (1999).

454 Barner, D., Libenson, A., Cheung, P. & Takasaki, M. Cross-linguistic relations between quantifiers and numerals in language acquisition: evidence from Japanese. *J. Exp. Child Psychol.* **103**, 421–440, doi:10.1016/j.jecp.2008.12.001 (2009).

455 Sarnecka, B. W., Kamenskaya, V. G., Yamana, Y., Ogura, T. & Yudovina, Y. B. From grammatical number to exact numbers: Early meanings of 'one', 'two', and 'three' in English, Russian, and Japanese. *Cognitive Psychology* **55**, 136–168, doi:10.1016/j.cogpsych.2006.09.001 (2007).

456 Almoammer, A. *et al.* Grammatical morphology as a source of early number word meanings. *Proc. Natl. Acad. Sci. U.S.A.* **110**, 18448–18453, doi:10.1073/pnas.1313652110 (2013).

457 Levine, S. C., Suriyakham, L. W., Rowe, M. L., Huttenlocher, J. & Gunderson, E. A. What counts in the development of young children's number knowledge? *Dev. Psychol.* **46**, 1309–1319, doi:10.1037/a0019671 (2010).

458 Spaepen, E., Coppola, M., Spelke, E. S., Carey, S. E. & Goldin-Meadow, S. Number without a language model. *Proc. Natl. Acad. Sci. U.S.A.* **108**, 3163–3168, doi:10.1073/pnas.1015975108 (2011).

459 Gunderson, E. A. & Levine, S. C. Some types of parent number talk count more than others: relations between parents' input and children's cardinal-number knowledge. *Dev. Sci.* **14**, 1021–1032, doi:10.1111/j.1467-7687.2011.01050.x (2011).

460 Andres, M., Di Luca, S. & Pesenti, M. Finger counting: the missing tool? *Behav. Brain Sci.* **31**, 642, doi:10.1017/s0140525x08005578 (2008).

461 Orban, G. A. *et al.* Mapping the parietal cortex of human and non-human primates. *Neuropsychologia* **44**, 2647–2667, doi:10.1016/j.neuropsychologia. 2005.11.001 (2006).

462 Rips, L. J., Bloomfield, A. & Asmuth, J. From numerical concepts to concepts of number. *Behav. Brain Sci.* **31**, 623, doi:10.1017/s0140525x08005566 (2008).

463 Tang, Y. Y. *et al.* Arithmetic processing in the brain shaped by cultures. *Proc. Natl. Acad. Sci. U.S.A.* **103**, 10775–10780, doi:10.1073/pnas.0604416103 (2006).

464 Ansari, D. Effects of development and enculturation on number represen-tation in the brain. *Nature Reviews Neuroscience* **9**, 278–291, doi:10.1038/nrn2334 (2008).

465 Diester, I. & Nieder, A. Complementary contributions of prefrontal neuron classes in abstract numerical categorization. *Journal of Neuroscience* **28**, 7737–7747, doi:10.1523/jneurosci.1347-08.2008 (2008).

466 Fias, W., Lammertyn, J., Caessens, B. & Orban, G. A. Processing of abstract ordinal knowledge in the horizontal segment of the intraparietal sulcus. *Journal of Neuroscience* **27**, 8952–8956, doi:10.1523/jneurosci.2076-07.2007 (2007).

467 Orban, G. A. *et al.* Mapping the parietal cortex of human and non-human primates. *Neuropsychologia* **44**, 2647–2667, doi:10.1016/j.neuropsychologia. 2005.11.001 (2006).

468 Miller, E. K., Nieder, A., Freedman, D. J. & Wallis, J. D. Neural correlates of categories and concepts. *Curr. Opin. Neurobiol.* **13**, 198–203, doi:10.1016/s0959-4388(03)00037-0 (2003).

469 Krinzinger, H. *et al.* The role of finger representations and saccades for number processing: an fMRI study in children. *Frontiers in Psychology* **2**, doi:10.3389/fpsyg.2011.00373 (2011).

470 Cantlon, J. F., Platt, M. L. & Brannon, E. M. Beyond the number domain. *Trends in Cognitive Sciences* **13**, 83–91, doi:10.1016/j.tics.2008.11.007.

471 Culham, J. C. & Kanwisher, N. G. Neuroimaging of cognitive functions in human parietal cortex. *Curr. Opin. Neurobiol.* **11**, 157–163, doi:10.1016/s0959-4388(00)00191-4 (2001).

472 Imbo, I., Vandierendonck, A. & Fias, W. Passive hand movements disrupt adults' counting strategies. *Frontiers in Psychology* **2**, 201, doi:10.3389/fpsyg. 2011.00201 (2011).

473 Klein, E., Moeller, K., Willmes, K., Nuerk, H.-C. & Domahs, F. The influ-ence of implicit hand-based representations on mental arithmetic. *Frontiers in Psychology* **2**, 197, doi:10.3389/fpsyg.2011.00197 (2011).

474 Domahs, F., Moeller, K., Huber, S., Willmes, K. & Nuerk, H. C. Embodied numerosity: implicit hand-based representations influence symbolic number processing across cultures. *Cognition* **116**, 251–266, doi:10.1016/j.cognition. 2010.05.007 (2010).

475 Gracia-Bafalluy, M. & Noel, M.-P. Does finger training increase young chil-dren's numerical performance? *Cortex* **44**, 368–375 (2008).

476 Moeller, K., Martignon, L., Wessolowski, S., Engel, J. & Nuerk, H.-C. Effects of finger counting on numerical development: the opposing views

of neurocognition and mathematics education. *Frontiers in Psychology* **2**, 328, doi:10.3389/fpsyg.2011.00328 (2011).

477 Barth, H., La Mont, K., Lipton, J. & Spelke, E. S. Abstract number and arithmetic in preschool children. *Proc. Natl. Acad. Sci. U.S.A.* **102**, 14116–14121, doi:10.1073/pnas.0505512102 (2005).

478 Berch, D. B., Foley, E. J., Hill, R. J. & Ryan, P. M. Extracting parity and magnitude from Arabic numerals: developmental changes in number processing and mental representation. *J. Exp. Child Psychol.* **74**, 286–308, doi:10.1006/jecp.1999.2518 (1999).

479 Soltesz, F., Szucs, D. & Szucs, L. Relationships between magnitude representation, counting and memory in 4- to 7-year-old children: a developmental study. *Behavioral and Brain Functions* **6**, 14, doi:10.1186/1744-9081-6-13 (2010).

480 Berteletti, I., Lucangeli, D., Piazza, M., Dehaene, S. & Zorzi, M. Numerical estimation in preschoolers. *Dev. Psychol.* **46**, 545–551, doi:10.1037/a0017887 (2010).

481 Siegler, R. S. & Booth, J. L. Development of numerical estimation in young children. *Child Development* **75**, 428–444, doi:10.1111/j.1467-8624.2004.00684.x (2004).

482 Halberda, J., Mazzocco, M. M. M. & Feigenson, L. Individual differences in non-verbal number acuity correlate with maths achievement. *Nature* **455**, 665-668, doi:10.1038/nature07246 (2008).

483 Gobel, S. M., Watson, S. E., Lervag, A. & Hulme, C. Children's arithmetic development: it is number knowledge, not the approximate number sense, that counts. *Psychological Science* **25**, 789–798, doi:10.1177/0956797613516471 (2014).

484 De Smedt, B., Noël, M.-P., Gilmore, C. & Ansari, D. How do symbolic and non-symbolic numerical magnitude processing skills relate to individual differences in children's mathematical skills? A review of evidence from brain and behavior. *Trends in Neuroscience and Education* **2**, 48–55, doi:dx.doi.org/10.1016/j.tine.2013.06.001 (2013).

485 Holloway, I. D. & Ansari, D. Mapping numerical magnitudes onto symbols: the numerical distance effect and individual differences in children's mathematics achievement. *J. Exp. Child Psychol.* **103**, 17–29, doi:10.1016/j.jecp.2008.04.001 (2009).

486 Siegler, R. S., Thompson, C. A. & Schneider, M. An integrated theory of whole number and fractions development. *Cognitive Psychology* **62**, 273–296, doi:10.1016/j.cogpsych.2011.03.001 (2011).

487 Butterworth, B. The development of arithmetical abilities. *Journal of Child Psychology and Psychiatry* **46**, 3–18, doi:10.1111/j.1469-7610.2005.00374.x (2005).

488 Kucian, K. *et al.* Mental number line training in children with developmental dyscalculia. *Neuroimage* **57**, 782–795, doi:10.1016/j.neuroimage.2011.01.070 (2011).

489 Hornstra, L., Denessen, E., Bakker, J., van den Bergh, L. & Voeten, M. Teacher attitudes toward dyslexia: effects on teacher expectations and the

academic achievement of students with dyslexia. *Journal of Learning Disabilities* **43**, 515–529, doi:10.1177/0022219409355479 (2010).

490 Delazer, M. *et al.* Learning complex arithmetic: an fMRI study. *Cognitive Brain Research* **18**, 76–88 (2003).

491 Bar-Matthews, M. *et al.* A high resolution and continuous isotopic speleothem record of paleoclimate and paleoenvironment from 90 to 53 ka from Pinnacle Point on the south coast of South Africa. *Quat. Sci. Rev.* **29**, 2131–2145, doi:10.1016/j.quascirev.2010.05.009 (2010).

492 d'Errico, F., Henshilwood, C., Vanhaeren, M. & van Niekerk, K. Nassarius kraussianus shell beads from Blombos Cave: evidence for symbolic behaviour in the Middle Stone Age. *J. Hum. Evol.* **48**, 3–24, doi:10.1016/j.jhevol. 2004.09.002 (2005).

493 Ambrose, S. H. Chronology of the later Stone Age and food production in East Africa. *Journal of Archaeological Science* **25**, 377–392, doi:10.1006/ jasc.1997.0277 (1998).

494 Kuhn, S. L. *et al.* The early Upper Paleolithic occupations at Ucagizli Cave (Hatay, Turkey). *J. Hum. Evol.* **56**, 87–113, doi:10.1016/j.jhevol.2008.07.014 (2009).

495 Adapted from Marshack, A. *Notation dans les Gravures du Paléolithique Supérieur* (Delmas/Don's Maps, 1970).

496 Jègues-Wolkiewiez, C. Aux racine de l'astronomie, ou l'ordre cache d'une paleolithique. *Antiquities Nationales* **37**, 43–62 (2005).

497 Overmann, K. A. Material scaffolds in numbers and time. *Cambridge Archaeological Journal* **23**, 19–39, doi:10.1017/s0959774313000024 (2013).

498 d'Errico, F. & Cacho, C. Notation versus decoration in the upper Palaeolithic: a case-study from Tossal de la Roca, Alicante, Spain. *Journal of Archaeological Science* **21**, 185–200, doi:dx.doi.org/10.1006/jasc.1994.1021 (1994).

499 Overmann, K. A., Wynn, T. & Coolidge, F. L. The prehistory of number concept. *Behav. Brain Sci.* **34**, 142–143, doi:10.1017/s0140525x10002189 (2011).

500 Epps, P., Bowern, C., Hansen, C. A., Hill, J. H. & Zentz, J. On numeral complexity in hunter-gatherer languages. *Linguistic Typology* **16**, 41–109, doi:10.1515/ lingty-2012-0002 (2012).

501 Caracuta, V. *et al.* The onset of faba bean farming in the Southern Levant. *Scientific Reports* **5**, 9, doi:10.1038/srep14370 (2015).

502 Lemmen, C. & Wirtz, K. W. On the sensitivity of the simulated European Neolithic transition to climate extremes. *Journal of Archaeological Science* **51**, 65–72, doi:10.1016/j.jas.2012.10.023 (2014).

503 Bettinger, R., Richerson, P. & Boyd, R. Constraints on the development of agriculture. *Curr. Anthropol.* **50**, 627–631, doi:10.1086/605359 (2009).

504 Kuijt, I. & Goring-Morris, N. Foraging, farming, and social complexity in the Pre-Pottery Neolithic of the Southern Levant: a review and synthesis. *Journal of World Prehistory* **16**, 361–440, doi:10.1023/a:1022973114090 (2002).

505 Schmandt-Besserat, D. *How writing came about* (University of Texas Press, 1996).

506 Schmandt-Besserat, D. in *The origins of writing* (ed. W. M. Senner), 27–41 (University of Nebraska Press, 1991).

507 Mullins, D. A., Whitehouse, H. & Atkinson, Q. D. The role of writing and recordkeeping in the cultural evolution of human cooperation. *J. Econ. Behav. Organ.* **90**, S141–S151, doi:10.1016/j.jebo.2012.12.017 (2013).

508 Coulmas, F. *Writing systems: An introduction to their linguistic analysis* (Cambridge University Press, 2003).

509 Woods, C. in *Visible language: Inventions of writing in the Ancient Middle East and beyond* (eds C. Woods, E. Teeter & G. Emberling), 33–84 (The Oriental Institute of the University of Chicago, 2015).

510 Adapted from Woods, C. *Visible language* (The Oriental Institute of the University of Chicago, 2015).

511 Li, X., Harbottle, G., Zhang, H. & Wnag, C. The earliest writing? Sign use in the seventh millennium BC at Jiahu, Henan Province, China. *Antiquity* **77**, 31–43 (2003).

512 Mann, C. C. Archaeology: unraveling khipu's secrets. *Science* **309**, 1008–1009, doi:10.1126/science.309.5737.1008 (2005).

513 Urton, G. Tying the archive in knots, or: dying to get into the archive in ancient Peru. *J. Soc. Arch.* **32**, 5–20, doi:10.1080/00379816.2011.563100 (2011).

514 Urton, G. & Brezine, C. J. Khipu accounting in ancient Peru. *Science* **309**, 1065–1067, doi:10.1126/science.1113426 (2005).

515 Changizi, M. A., Zhang, Q., Ye, H. & Shimojo, S. The structures of letters and symbols throughout human history are selected to match those found in objects in natural scenes. *Am. Nat.* **167**, E117–E139, doi:10.1086/502806 (2006).

516 Ashby, J., & Rayner, K. in *Cognitive neuroscience: The good, the bad, and the ugly* (eds S. Della Sala & M. Anderson), 61–83 (Oxford University Press, 2012).

517 Dehaene, S. & Cohen, L. The unique role of the visual word form area in reading. *Trends in Cognitive Sciences* **15**, 254–262, doi:10.1016/j.tics.2011.04.003 (2011).

518 Barquero, L. A., Davis, N. & Cutting, L. E. Neuroimaging of reading intervention: a systematic review and activation likelihood estimate meta-analysis. *PLOS One* **9**, 16, doi:10.1371/journal.pone.0083668 (2014).

519 Price, C. J. A review and synthesis of the first 20 years of PET and fMRI studies of heard speech, spoken language and reading. *Neuroimage* **62**, 816–847, doi:10.1016/j.neuroimage.2012.04.062 (2012).

520 Shaywitz, S. E. & Shaywitz, B. A. Paying attention to reading: the neurobiology of reading and dyslexia. *Dev. Psychopathol.* **20**, 1329–1349, doi:10.1017/s0954579408000631 (2008).

521 Ehri, L. C. in Learning and teaching reading, *British Journal of Educational Psychology Monograph* (eds R. Stainthorp & P. Tomlinson) (2002).

522 Jorm, A. F. & Share, D. L. Phonological recoding and reading acquisition. *Appl. Psycholinguist.* **4**, 103–147, doi:10.1017/s0142716400004380 (1983).

523 Share, D. L. Phonological recoding and self-teaching: sine-qua-non of reading acquisition. *Cognition* **55**, 151–218, doi:10.1016/0010-0277(94)00645-2 (1995).

524 Turkeltaub, P. E., Gareau, L., Flowers, D. L., Zeffiro, T. A. & Eden, G. F. Development of neural mechanisms of reading. *Nature Neuroscience* **6**, 767–773 (2003).

525 Van Ettinger-Veenstra, H., Ragnehed, M., McAllister, A., Lundberg, P. & Engstrom, M. Right-hemispheric cortical contributions to language ability in healthy adults. *Brain and Language* **120**, 395–400, doi:10.1016/j.bandl.2011.10.002 (2012).

526 Horowitz-Kraus, T. *et al.* Right is not always wrong: DTI and fMRI evidence for the reliance of reading comprehension on language-comprehension networks in the right hemisphere. *Brain Imaging and Behavior* **9**, 19–31, doi:10.1007/s11682-014-9341-9 (2015).

527 Howard-Jones, P. A., Blakemore, S. J., Samuel, E., Summers, I. R. & Claxton, G. Semantic divergence and creative story generation: an fMRI investigation. *Cognitive Brain Research* **25**, 240–250 (2005).

528 Kolb, B. & Whishaw, I. *Fundamentals of human neuropsychology*, 3rd edn (Freeman, 1990).

529 Geake, J. G. Neuromythologies in education. *Educational Research* **50**, 123–133 (2008).

530 Welcome, S. E. & Joanisse, M. F. Individual differences in white matter anatomy predict dissociable components of reading skill in adults. *Neuroimage* **96**, 261–275, doi:10.1016/j.neuroimage.2014.03.069 (2014).

531 Sylva, K., Melhuish, E., Sammons, P., Siraj-Blatchford, I. & Taggart, B. Effective pre-school education: a longitudinal study funded by the DfES (1997–2004) (Institute of Education, Nottingham, 2004).

532 Diamond, M. C. *et al.* Rat cortical morphology following crowded-enriched living conditions. *Experimental Neurology* **96**, 241–247 (1987).

533 Greenough, W. T., Black, J. E. & Wallace, C. S. Experience and brain development. *Child Development* **58**, 539–559 (1987). [Quoted material can be found on p. 246.]

534 Howard-Jones, P. A., Washbrook, E. V. & Meadows, S. The timing of educational investment: a neuroscientific perspective. *Developmental Cognitive Neuroscience* **2**, Supplement 1, S18–S29, doi:10.1016/j.dcn.2011.11.002 (2012).

535 Blakemore, S. J. Imaging brain development: the adolescent brain. *Neuroimage* **61**, 397–406, doi:10.1016/j.neuroimage.2011.11.080 (2012).

536 Knoll, L. J. *et al.* A window of opportunity for cognitive training in adolescence. *Psychological Science* **27**, 1620–1631 (2016).

537 Hasson, U., Levy, I., Behrmann, M., Hendler, T. & Malach, R. Eccentricity bias as an organizing principle for human high-order object areas. *Neuron* **34**, 479–490, doi:10.1016/s0896-6273(02)00662-1 (2002).

538 Szwed, M., Cohen, L., Qiao, E. & Dehaene, S. The role of invariant line junctions in object and visual word recognition. *Vision Res.* **49**, 718–725, doi:10.1016/j.visres.2009.01.003 (2009).

539 Epelbaum, S. *et al.* Pure alexia as a disconnection syndrome: new diffusion imaging evidence for an old concept. *Cortex* **44**, 962–974, doi:10.1016/j.cortex.2008.05.003 (2008).

540 Pinel, P. & Dehaene, S. Beyond hemispheric dominance: brain regions underlying the joint lateralization of language and arithmetic to the left hemisphere. *Journal of Cognitive Neuroscience* **22**, 48–66, doi:10.1162/jocn.2009.21184 (2010).

541 Dehaene, S., Cohen, L., Morais, J. & Kolinsky, R. Illiterate to literate: behavioural and cerebral changes induced by reading acquisition. *Nature Reviews Neuroscience* **16**, 234–274, doi:10.1038/nrn3924 (2015).

542 Dehaene, S. *et al.* How learning to read changes the cortical networks for vision and language. *Science* **330**, 1359–1364, doi:10.1126/science.1194140 (2010).

543 Pinel, P. *et al.* Genetic and environmental influences on the visual word form and fusiform face areas. *Cerebral Cortex* **25**, 2478–2493, doi:10.1093/cercor/bhu048 (2015).

544 Ventura, P. *et al.* Literacy acquisition reduces the influence of automatic holistic processing of faces and houses. *Neurosci. Lett.* **554**, 105–109, doi:10.1016/j.neulet.2013.08.068 (2013).

545 Lachmann, T. & van Leeuwen, C. Paradoxical enhancement of letter recognition in developmental dyslexia. *Developmental Neuropsychology* **31**, 61–77, doi:10.1207/s15326942dn3101_4 (2007).

546 Pegado, F., Nakamura, K. & Hannagan, T. How does literacy break mirror invariance in the visual system? *Frontiers in Psychology* **5**, doi:10.3389/fpsyg.2014.00703 (2014).

547 Andoni Dunabeitia, J., Dimitropoulou, M., Estevez, A. & Carreiras, M. The influence of reading expertise in mirror-letter perception: evidence from beginning and expert readers. *Mind Brain and Education* **7**, 124–135, doi:10.1111/mbe.12017 (2013).

548 Kolinsky, R. *et al.* Enantiomorphy through the looking glass: literacy effects on mirror-image discrimination. *J. Exp. Psychol.-Gen.* **140**, 210–238, doi:10.1037/a0022168 (2011).

549 Richlan, F. Developmental dyslexia: dysfunction of a left hemisphere reading network. *Front. Hum. Neurosci.* **6**, doi:10.3389/fnhum.2012.00120 (2012).

550 Pugh, K. R. *et al.* Functional neuroimaging studies of reading and reading disability (developmental dyslexia). *Mental Retardation and Developmental Disabilities Research Reviews* **6**, 207–213, doi:10.1002/1098-2779(2000)6:3<207::aid-mrdd8>3.0.co;2-p (2000).

551 Goswami, U. Sensory theories of developmental dyslexia: three challenges for research. *Nature Reviews Neuroscience* **16**, 43–54, doi:10.1038/nrn3836 (2015).

552 Simos, P. G. *et al.* Dyslexia-specific brain activation profile becomes normal following successful remedial training. *Neurology* **58**, 1203–1213 (2002).

553 Temple, E. *et al.* Neural deficits in children with dyslexia ameliorated by behavioral remediation: evidence from functional MRI. *Proc. Natl. Acad. Sci. U.S.A.* **100**, 2860–2865, doi:10.1073/pnas.0030098100 (2003).

554 Shaywitz, B. A. *et al.* Development of left occipitotemporal systems for skilled reading in children after a phonologically-based intervention. *Biological Psychiatry* **55**, 926–933 (2004).

555 Aylward, E. H. *et al.* Instructional treatment associated with changes in brain activation in children with dyslexia. *Neurology* **61**, 212–219 (2003).

556 Yamada, Y. *et al.* Emergence of the neural network for reading in five-year old beginning readers of different levels of pre-literacy abilities: an fMRI study. *NeuroImage* **57**, 704–713, doi:10.1016/j.neuroimage.2010.10.057 (2011).

557 Elliott, J. G. & Grigorenko, E. L. The end of dyslexia? *Psychologist* **27**, 576–580 (2014).

558 Thomas, M. S. C. On hermit crabs and humans. *Dev. Sci.* **16**, 314–316, doi:10.1111/desc.12031 (2013).

559 Dehaene, S., Spelke, E., Pinel, P., Stanescu, R. & Tsivkin, S. Sources of mathematical thinking: behavioral and brain-imaging evidence. *Science* **284**, 970–974 (1999).

560 Chen, Y. L., Yanke, J. & Campbell, J. I. D. Language-specific memory for everyday arithmetic facts in Chinese-English bilinguals. *Psychol. Bull. Rev.* **23**, 526–532, doi:10.3758/s13423-015-0920-6 (2016).

561 Salillas, E. & Carreiras, M. Core number representations are shaped by language. *Cortex* **52**, 1–11, doi:10.1016/j.cortex.2013.12.009 (2014).

562 Guha, S. & Sudha, A. Origin and history of value education in India: understanding the ancient Indian educational system. *Indian Journal of Applied Research* **VI** (2016).

563 Wang, X. X. Formation and establishment of study of Confucian classics as educational core in ancient China. *M&D Forum*, 203–206 (2013).

564 EFA. *2015 global monitoring report: Education for all 2000–2015: Achievements and challenges* (UNESCO, 2015).

565 Kosmidis, M. H., Zafiri, M. & Politimou, N. Literacy versus formal schooling: influence on working memory. *Arch. Clin. Neuropsychol.* **26**, 575–582, doi:10.1093/arclin/acr063 (2011).

566 Kosmidis, M. H., Tsapkini, K. & Folia, V. Lexical processing in illiteracy: effect of literacy or education? *Cortex* **42**, 1021–1027, doi:10.1016/s0010-9452(08)70208-9 (2006).

567 Ardila, A., Ostrosky-Solis, F., Rosselli, M. & Gomez, C. Age-related cognitive decline during normal aging: the complex effect of education. *Arch. Clin. Neuropsychol.* **15**, 495–513, doi:10.1016/s0887-6177(99)00040-2 (2000).

568 Ostrosky-Solis, F., Ardila, A., Rosselli, M., Lopez-Arango, G. & Uriel-Mendoza, V. Neuropsychological test performance in illiterate subjects. *Arch. Clin. Neuropsychol.* **13**, 645–660, doi:10.1016/s0887-6177(97)00094-2 (1998).

569 Reis, A., Guerreiro, M. & Petersson, K. M. A sociodemographic and neuropsychological characterization of an illiterate population. *Appl. Neuropsychol.* **10**, 191–204, doi:10.1207/s15324826an1004_1 (2003).

570 Ardila, A. *et al.* Illiteracy: the neuropsychology of cognition without reading. *Arch. Clin. Neuropsychol.* **25**, 689–712, doi:10.1093/arclin/acq079 (2010).

571 Ciborowski, I. J. in *Perspectives in cross-cultural psychology* (eds A. J. Marsella, R. G. Tharp & I. J. Ciborowski), 101–116 (Academic Press, 1979).

572 Nitrini, R. *et al.* Performance of illiterate and literate nondemented elderly subjects in two tests of long-term memory. *J. Int. Neuropsychol. Soc.* **10**, 634–638, doi:10.1017/s1355617704104062 (2004).

573 Yassuda, M. S. *et al.* Neuropsychological profile of Brazilian older adults with heterogeneous educational backgrounds. *Arch. Clin. Neuropsychol.* **24**, 71–79, doi:10.1093/arclin/acp009 (2009).

574 Cornelius, S. W. & Caspi, A. Everyday problem-solving in adulthood and old-age. *Psychol. Aging* **2**, 144–153, doi:10.1037//0882-7974.2.2.144 (1987).

575 Reyes-Garcia, V. *et al.* Schooling, local knowledge and working memory: a study among three contemporary hunter-gatherer societies. *PLOS One* **11**, 18, doi:10.1371/journal.pone.0145265 (2016).

576 Erikson, R. & Jonsson, J. O. in *Can education be equalized?* (eds R. Erikson & J. O. Jonsson) (Westview, 1996).

577 Shavit, Y. & Müller, W. *From school to work: A comparative study of educational qualifications and occupational destinations* (Clarendon Press, 1998).

578 Fusco, A., Guio, A.-C. & Marlier, E. in *Income and living conditions in Europe* (eds A. B. Marlier & E. Atkinson), 133–153 (Office for Official Publications of the European Communities (OPOCE), 2010).

579 Gesthuizen, M. & Scheepers, P. Economic vulnerability among low-educated europeans resource, composition, labour market and welfare state influences. *Acta Sociol.* **53**, 247–267, doi:10.1177/0001699310374491 (2010).

580 Cutler, D. M. & Lleras-Muney, A. Understanding differences in health behaviors by education. *J. Health Econ.* **29**, 1–28, doi:10.1016/j.jhealeco.2009.10.003 (2010).

581 Then, F. S., Luck, T., Angermeyer, M. C. & Riedel-Heller, S. G. Education as protector against dementia, but what exactly do we mean by education? *Age Ageing* **45**, 523–528, doi:10.1093/ageing/afw049 (2016).

582 Oreopoulos, P. & Salvanes, K. G. Priceless: The nonpecuniary benefits of schooling. *J. Econ. Perspect.* **25**, 159–184, doi:10.1257/jep.25.1.159 (2011).

583 Reinke, E. C. Quintilian lighted the way. *Class. Bull.* **51**, 65–71 (1975).

584 Darwin, C. R. Letter to Mrs. Emily Talbot on the mental and bodily development of infants: report of the secretary of the department. *Journal of Social Science, containing the Transactions of the American Association* **15**, 5–8 (1882).

585 Haeckel, E. H. P. A. *Generelle Morphologie Der Organismen: Allgemeine Grundzuge Der Organischen Formen-Wissenschaft, Mechanisch Begrundet Durch Die Von Charles Darwin Reformirte Descendenz-Theorie* (G. Reimer, 1866).

586 Pérez, B. *The first three years of childhood* (Swan Sonnenschein & Co, 1885).

587 Choudhury, S. Culturing the adolescent brain: what can neuroscience learn from anthropology? *Social Cognitive and Affective Neuroscience* **5**, 159–167, doi:10.1093/scan/nsp030 (2010).

588 Hall, G. S. *Adolescence: Its psychology and its relations to physiology, anthropology, sociology, sex, crime, religion and education* (D. Appleton and Company, 1904).

589 Kalinka, A. T. & Tomancak, P. The evolution of early animal embryos: conservation or divergence? *Trends Ecol. Evol.* **27**, 385–393, doi:dx.doi.org/10.1016/j.tree.2012.03.007 (2012).

590 Koops, W. No developmental psychology without recapitulation theory. *European Journal of Developmental Psychology* **12**, 630–639, doi:10.1080/174056 29.2015.1078234 (2015).

591 Pass, S. *Parallel paths to constructivism: Jean Piaget and Lev Vygotsky* (Information Age Publishing, 2004).

592 Doman, C. H. *The diagnosis and treatment of speech and reading problems* (Thomas, 1968).

593 Chapanis, N. P. in *Brain dysfunction in children: etiology, diagnosis, and management* (ed. P. Black), 265–280 (Raven Press, 1982).

594 Cohen, H. J., Birch, H. G. & Taft, L. T. Some considerations for evaluating the Doman-Delecato "patterning" method. *Pediatrics* **45**, 302–314 (1970).

595 Cummins, R. A. *The neurologically impaired child: Doman-Delacato techniques reappraised* (Croom Helm, 1988).

596 Robbins, M. P. & Glass, G. V. in *Educational therapy* (ed. J. Hellmuth), 323–377 (Special Child Publications, 1968).

597 Ziring, P. R. *et al.* Learning disabilities, dyslexia, and vision: A subject review. *Pediatrics* **103**, 1217–1219 (1998).

598 Dennison, P. E. *Switching on: A guide to Edu-Kinesthetics* (Edu-Kinesthetics, 1981).

599 Dennison, P. E. & Dennison, G. E. *Brain gym teacher's edition: Revised* (Edu-Kinesthetics, 1994).

600 Hyatt, K. J. Brain gym: building stronger brains or wishful thinking? *Remedial and Special Education* **28**, 117–124 (2007).

601 Howard-Jones, P. A. Neuroscience and education: myths and messages. *Nature Reviews Neuroscience* **15**, 817–824 (2014).

602 MacLean, P. *A mind of three minds: Educating the triune brain, 77th year book of the national society of the study of education* (University of Chicago Press, 1978).

603 Nummela, R. M. & Rosengren, T. M. The triune brain: a new paradigm for education. *Journal of Humanistic Counseling, Education & Development* **24**, 98–103 (1986).

604 Krubitzer, L. A. & Seelke, A. M. H. Cortical evolution in mammals: the bane and beauty of phenotypic variability. *Proc. Natl. Acad. Sci. U.S.A.* **109**, 10647–10654, doi:10.1073/pnas.1201891109 (2012).

605 Narvaez, D. Triune ethics: the neurobiological roots of our multiple moralities. *New Ideas Psychol.* **26**, 95–119, doi:10.1016/j.newideapsych.2007.07.008 (2008).

606 IPSOS. *Supreme being, the afterlife, and evolution*, www.ipsos-na.com/news-polls/pressrelease.aspx?id=5217 (2011).

607 Paz-y-Miño-C, G. & Espinosa, A. Educators of prospective teachers hesitate to embrace evolution due to deficient understanding of science/evolution and high religiosity. *Evolution: Education and Outreach* **5**, 139–162, doi:10.1007/s12052-011-0383-9 (2012).

608 Paz-Y-Mino-C, G. & Espinosa, A. Introduction: why people do not accept evolution: using protistan diversity to promote evolution literacy. *Journal of Eukaryotic Microbiology* **59**, 101–104, doi:10.1111/j.1550-7408.2011.00604.x (2012).

609 Weisberg, D. S., Keil, F. C., Goodstein, J., Rawson, E. & Gray, J. The seductive lure of neuroscience explanations. *Journal of Cognitive Neuroscience* **20**, 470–477 (2008).

610 Cosmides, L. The logic of social exchange: has natural selection shaped how humans reason? Studies with the Wason selection task. *Cognition* **31**, 187–276, doi:10.1016/0010-0277(89)90023-1 (1989).

611 Buss, D. M., Larsen, R. J., Westen, D. & Semmelroth, J. Sex-differences in jealousy: evolution, physiology and psychology. *Psychological Science* **3**, 251–255, doi:10.1111/j.1467-9280.1992.tb00038.x (1992).

612 Buller, D. J. Evolutionary psychology: the emperor's new paradigm. *Trends in Cognitive Sciences* **9**, 277–283, doi:10.1016/j.tics.2005.04.003 (2005).

613 Almor, A. & Sloman, S. A. Reasoning versus text processing in the Wason selection task: a nondeontic perspective on perspective effects. *Mem. Cogn.* **28**, 1060–1070, doi:10.3758/bf03209354 (2000).

614 Stewart-Williams, S. & Thomas, A. G. The ape that thought it was a peacock: does evolutionary psychology exaggerate human sex differences? *Psychological Inquiry* **24**, 137–168, doi:10.1080/1047840x.2013.804899 (2013).

615 Harris, C. R. Humans, deer, and sea dragons: how evolutionary psychology has misconstrued human sex differences. *Psychological Inquiry* **24**, 195–201, doi: 10.1080/1047840x.2013.817323 (2013).

616 Harris, C. R. Sexual and romantic jealousy in heterosexual and homosexual adults. *Psychological Science* **13**, 7–12, doi:10.1111/1467-9280.00402 (2002).

617 Harris, C. R. Factors associated with jealousy over real and imagined infidelity: an examination of the social-cognitive and evolutionary psychology perspectives. *Psychology of Women Quarterly* **27**, 319–329, doi:10.1111/1471-6402.00112 (2003).

618 DeSteno, D., Bartlett, M. Y., Braverman, J. & Salovey, P. Sex differences in jealousy: evolutionary mechanism or artifact of measurement? *J. Pers. Soc. Psychol.* **83**, 1103–1116, doi:10.1037//0022-3514.83.5.1103 (2002).

619 Sheets, V. L. & Wolfe, M. D. Sexual jealousy in heterosexuals, lesbians, and gays. *Sex Roles* **44**, 255-276, doi:10.1023/a:1010996631863 (2001).

620 Buller, D. J. *Adapting minds: Evolutionary psychology and the persistent quest for human nature* (MIT Press, 2005).

621 Gould, S. J. & Lewontin, R. C. *The spandrels of San Marco and the panglossian paradigm: A critique of the adaptationist programme* (MIT Press, 1994).

622 Brinkmann, S. Can we save Darwin from evolutionary psychology? *Nord. Psychol.* **63**, 50–67, doi:10.1027/1901-2276/a000039 (2011). [Quoted material can be found on p. 64.]

623 Panksepp, J. & Panksepp, J. The seven sins of evolutionary psychology. *Evolution and Cognition* **6**, 108–131 (2000). [Quoted material can be found on p. 113.]

624 Geary, D. C. An evolutionarily informed education science. *Educational Psychologist* **43**, 179–195, doi:10.1080/00461520802392133 (2008).

625 Geary, D. C. Evolution and education. *Psicothema* **22**, 35–40 (2010).

626 Halpern, D. F. How much can evolutionary psychology inform the educational sciences? *Educational Psychologist* **43**, 203–205, doi:10.1080/004615 20802392224 (2008).

627 Ellis, G. F. R. Commentary on "an evolutionarily informed education science" by David C. Geary. *Educational Psychologist* **43**, 206–213, doi:10.1080/ 00461520802392216 (2008).

628 Izuma, K., Saito, D. N. & Sadato, N. Processing of social and monetary rewards in the human striatum. *Neuron* **58**, 284–294, doi:10.1016/j.neuron.2008.03.020 (2008).

629 Howard-Jones, P. A., Jay, T., Mason, A. & Jones, H. Gamification of learning deactivates the default mode network. *Frontiers in Psychology* **6**, 16, doi:10.3389/fpsyg.2015.01891 (2016).

630 Knutson, B., Adams, C. M., Fong, G. W. & Hommer, D. Anticipation of monetary reward selectively recruits nucleus accumbens. *Journal of Neuroscience* **21**, 1–5 (2001).

631 Farooqi, I. S. *et al.* Leptin regulates striatal regions and human eating behavior. *Science* **317**, 1355–1355, doi:10.1126/science.1144599 (2007).

632 Koepp, M. J. *et al.* Evidence for striatal dopamine release during a video game. *Nature* **393**, 266–268 (1998).

633 Schomaker, J. & Meeter, M. Short- and long-lasting consequences of novelty, deviance and surprise on brain and cognition. *Neurosci. Biobehav. Rev.* **55**, 268–279, doi:10.1016/j.neubiorev.2015.05.002 (2015).

634 Min Jeong, K. *et al.* The wick in the candle of learning: epistemic curiosity activates reward circuitry and enhances memory. *Psychological Science (0956–7976)* **20**, 963–973, doi:10.1111/j.1467-9280.2009.02402.x (2009).

635 Furukawa, E. *et al.* Abnormal striatal BOLD Responses to reward anticipation and reward delivery in ADHD. *PLOS One* **9**, 9, doi:10.1371/journal.pone.0089129 (2014).

636 Gaastra, G. F., Groen, Y., Tucha, L. & Tucha, O. The effects of classroom interventions on off-task and disruptive classroom behavior in children with symptoms of attention-deficit/hyperactivity disorder: a meta-analytic review. *PLOS One* **11**, 19, doi:10.1371/journal.pone.0148841 (2016).

637 Gallese, V. The roots of empathy: the shared manifold hypothesis and the neural basis of intersubjectivity. *Psychopathology* **36**, 171–180, doi:10.1159/000072786 (2003).

638 Gallese, V., Eagle, M. N. & Migone, P. Intentional attunement: mirror neurons and the neural underpinnings of interpersonal relations. *J. Am. Psychoanal. Assoc.* **55**, 131–176 (2007).

639 Wicker, B. *et al.* Both of us disgusted in my insula: the common neural basis of seeing and feeling disgust. *Neuron* **40**, 655–664, doi:dx.doi.org/10.1016/S0896-6273(03)00679-2 (2003).

640 Beilock, S. L., Gunderson, E. A., Ramirez, G. & Levine, S. C. Female teachers' math anxiety affects girls' math achievement. *Proc. Natl. Acad. Sci. U.S.A.* **107**, 1860–1863, doi:10.1073/pnas.0910967107 (2010).

641 Ker, H. W. The impacts of student-, teacher- and school-level factors on mathematics achievement: an exploratory comparative investigation of Singaporean students and the USA students. *Educational Psychology* **36**, 254–276, doi:10.1080/01443410.2015.1026801 (2016).

642 Inoue, S. & Matsuzawa, T. Working memory of numerals in chimpanzees. *Curr. Biol.* **17**, R1004-R1005, doi:10.1016/j.cub.2007.10.027.

643 Doherty-Sneddon, G., Phelps, F. G. & Calderwood, L. Gaze aversion during children's transient knowledge and learning. *Cogn. Instr.* **27**, 225–238, doi:10.1080/07370000903014329 (2009).

644 Olson, D. R. & Bruner, J. S. in *The handbook of education and human development* (eds D. R. Olson & N. Torrance), 9–27 (Blackwell, 1996).

645 Haim, O., Strauss, S. & Ravid, D. Relations between EFL teachers' formal knowledge of grammar and their in-action mental models of children's

minds and learning. *Teaching and Teacher Education* **20**, 861–880, doi:10.1016/j.tate.2004.09.007 (2004).

646 Mevorach, M. & Strauss, S. Teacher educators' in-action mental models in different teaching situations. *Teachers and Teaching* **18**, 25–41, doi:10.1080/13 540602.2011.622551 (2012).

647 Brod, G., Werkle-Bergner, M. & Shing, Y. L. The influence of prior knowledge on memory: a developmental cognitive neuroscience perspective. *Front. Behav. Neurosci.* **7**, 13, doi:10.3389/fnbeh.2013.00139 (2013).

648 Shing, Y. L. & Brod, G. Effects of prior knowledge on memory: implications for education. *Mind, Brain, and Education* **10**, 153–161, doi:10.1111/mbe.12110 (2016).

649 Bruinsma, Y., Koegel, R. L. & Koegel, L. K. Joint attention and children with autism: a review of the literature. *Mental Retardation and Developmental Disabilities Research Reviews* **10**, 169–175, doi:10.1002/mrdd.20036 (2004).

650 Charman, T. *et al.* Testing joint attention, imitation, and play as infancy precursors to language and theory of mind. *Cogn. Dev.* **15**, 481–498, doi:10.1016/s0885-2014(01)00037-5 (2000).

651 Dawson, G. *et al.* Neurocognitive function and joint attention ability in young children with autism spectrum disorder versus developmental delay. *Child Development* **73**, 345–358, doi:10.1111/1467-8624.00411 (2002).

652 Tomasello, M. & Farrar, M. J. Joint attention and early language. *Child Development* **57**, 1454–1463, doi:10.1111/j.1467-8624.1986.tb00470.x (1986).

653 Craik, F. I. M. & Lockhart, R. S. Levels of processing: framework for memory research. *Journal of Verbal Learning and Verbal Behavior* **11**, 671–684, doi:10.1016/s0022-5371(72)80001-x (1972).

654 McDaniel, M. A., Roediger, H. L. & McDermott, K. B. Generalizing test-enhanced learning from the laboratory to the classroom. *Psychon. Bull. Rev.* **14**, 200–206, doi:10.3758/bf03194052 (2007).

655 Roediger, H. L. & Karpicke, J. D. Test-enhanced learning: taking memory tests improves long-term retention. *Psychological Science* **17**, 249–255, doi:10.1111/j.1467-9280.2006.01693.x (2006).

656 Rohrer, D. & Pashler, H. Recent research on human learning challenges conventional instructional strategies. *Educational Researcher* **39**, 406–412, doi:10.3102/0013189x10374770 (2010).

657 Campbell, J. & Mayer, R. E. Questioning as an instructional method: does it affect learning from lectures? *Appl. Cogn. Psychol.* **23**, 747–759, doi:10.1002/acp.1513 (2009).

658 Johnson, C. I. & Mayer, R. E. A testing effect with multimedia learning. *Journal of Educational Psychology* **101**, 621–629, doi:10.1037/a0015183 (2009).

659 McDaniel, M. A., Agarwal, P. K., Huelser, B. J., McDermott, K. B. & Roediger, H. L. Test-enhanced learning in a middle school science classroom: the effects of quiz frequency and placement. *Journal of Educational Psychology* **103**, 399–414, doi:10.1037/a0021782 (2011).

660 Karpicke, J. D. & Blunt, J. R. Retrieval practice produces more learning than elaborative studying with concept mapping. *Science* **331**, 772–775, doi:10.1126/science.1199327 (2011).

661 Wirebring, L. K. *et al.* Lesser neural pattern similarity across repeated tests is associated with better long-term memory retention. *Journal of Neuroscience* **35**, 9595–9602, doi:10.1523/jneurosci.3550-14.2015 (2015).

662 Zimmer, H. D. & Cohen, R. L. in *Memory for action: A distinct form of episodic memory* (eds H. D. Zimmer *et al.*) (Oxford University Press, 2001).

663 Engelkamp, J. Some studies on the internal structure of propositions. *Psychol. Res.-Psychol. Forsch.* **41**, 355–371, doi:10.1007/bf00308880 (1980).

664 Engelkamp, J. & Krumnacker, H. The imaginal and motor processes as performance recall influences of verbal material. *Zeitschrift Fur Experimentelle Und Angewandte Psychologie* **27**, 511–533 (1980).

665 Engelkamp, J. & Zimmer, H. D. Motor program information as a separable memory unit. *Psychol. Res.-Psychol. Forsch.* **46**, 283–299, doi:10.1007/bf00308889 (1984).

666 Backman, L. & Nilsson, L. G. Prerequisites for lack of age-differences in memory performance. *Experimental Aging Research* **11**, 67–73 (1985).

667 Mimura, M. *et al.* Memory for subject performed tasks in patients with Korsak off syndrome. *Cortex* **34**, 297–303, doi:10.1016/s0010-9452(08)70757-3 (1998).

668 Karlsson, T. *et al.* Memory improvement at different stages of Alzheimers disease. *Neuropsychologia* **27**, 737–742, doi:10.1016/0028-3932(89)90119-x (1989).

669 Macedonia, M. & Mueller, K. Exploring the neural representation of novel words learned through enactment in a word recognition task. *Frontiers in Psychology* **7**, 14, doi:10.3389/fpsyg.2016.00953 (2016).

670 Fischer, U., Moeller, K., Bientzle, M., Cress, U. & Nuerk, H.-C. Sensorimotor spatial training of number magnitude representation. *Psychon. Bull. Rev.* **18**, 177–183, doi:10.3758/s13423-010-0031-3 (2011).

671 Johnson-Glenberg, M. C., Birchfield, D. A., Tolentino, L. & Koziupa, T. Collaborative embodied learning in mixed reality motion-capture environments: two science studies. *Journal of Educational Psychology* **106**, 86–104, doi:10.1037/a0034008 (2014).

672 Galland, B. *et al.* Sleep disordered breathing and academic performance: a meta-analysis. *Pediatrics* **136**, E934-E946, doi:10.1542/peds.2015-1677 (2015).

673 Curcio, G., Ferrara, M. & De Gennaro, L. Sleep loss, learning capacity and academic performance. *Sleep Medicine Reviews* **10**, 323–337, doi:10.1016/j.smrv.2005.11.001 (2006).

674 Kirby, M., Maggi, S. & D'Angiulli, A. School start times and the sleep-wake cycle of adolescents: a review and critical evaluation of available evidence. *Educational Researcher* **40**, 56–61, doi:10.3102/0013189x11402323 (2011).

675 Howard-Jones, P. *et al.* The principles and practices of educational neuroscience: commentary on Bowers (2016). *Psychological Review* (in press).

676 Dehaene, S. *Reading in the brain* (Viking Penguin, 2009).

677 Hausfather, Z. *et al.* Assessing recent warming using instrumentally homogeneous sea surface temperature records. *Sci. Adv.* **3**, 13, doi:10.1126/sciadv.1601207 (2017).

678 Graph adapted from Goddard Institute for Space Studies Surface Temperature Analysis: https://data.giss.nasa.gov/gistemp.

679 Ceballos, G. *et al*. Accelerated modern human-induced species losses: entering the sixth mass extinction. *Sci. Adv*. **1**, doi:10.1126/sciadv.1400253 (2015).

680 Bulletin of the Atomic Scientists. *It is two and a half minutes to midnight* (2017). http://thebulletin.org/clock/2017.

681 Merrill, M. A. The significance of IQs on the revised Stanford-Binet scales. *Journal of Educational Psychology* **29**, 641–651, doi:10.1037/h0057523 (1938).

682 Tuddenham, R. D. Soldier intelligence in World Wars I and II. *American Psychologist* **3**, 54–56, doi:10.1037/h0054962 (1948).

683 Pietschnig, J. & Voracek, M. One century of global IQ gains: a formal meta-analysis of the Flynn Effect (1909–2013). *Perspect. Psychol. Sci*. **10**, 282–306, doi:10.1177/1745691615577701 (2015).

684 Trut, L. Early canid domestication: the farm-fox experiment. *American Scientist* **87**, doi:10.1511/1999.2.160 (1999).

685 Laland, K. N., Odling-Smee, J. & Myles, S. How culture shaped the human genome: bringing genetics and the human sciences together. *Nature Reviews Genetics* **11**, 137–148, doi:10.1038/nrg2734 (2010).

686 Livingstone, F. B. Anthropological implications of sickle-cell distribution in West Africa. *American Anthropologist* **60**, 533–562 (1958).

687 Durham, W. H. *Co-evolution: Genes, culture and human diversity* (Stanford University Press, 1991).

688 Hawley, W. A., Reiter, P., Copeland, R. S., Pumpuni, C. B. & Craig, G. B. Aedes albopictus in North America: probable introduction in used tires from Northern Asia. *Science* **236**, 1114–1116 (1987).

689 Rozsa, L. The rise of non-adaptive intelligence in humans under pathogen pressure. *Medical Hypotheses* **70**, 685–690, doi:10.1016/j.mehy.2007.06.028 (2008).

690 Evans, P. D. *et al*. Microcephalin, a gene regulating brain size, continues to evolve adaptively in humans. *Science* **309**, 1717–1720, doi:10.1126/science.1113722 (2005).

691 Mekel-Bobrov, N. *et al*. Ongoing adaptive evolution of ASPM, a brain size determinant in Homo sapiens. *Science* **309**, 1720–1722, doi:10.1126/science.1116815 (2005).

692 Balter, M. Are human brains still evolving? Brain genes show signs of selection. *Science* **309**, 1662–1663, doi:10.1126/science.309.5741.1662 (2005).

693 Rindermann, H. The g-factor of international cognitive ability comparisons: the homogeneity of results in PISA, TIMSS, PIRLS and IQtests across nations. *European Journal of Personality* **21**, 667–706 (2007).

694 Rindermann, H. The big G-factor of national cognitive ability. *European Journal of Personality* **21**, 767–787 (2007).

695 Fatemi, S. H., Folsom, T. D., Reutiman, T. J. & Sidwell, R. W. Viral regulation of aquaporin 4, connexin 43, microcephalin and nucleolin. *Schizophrenia Research* **98**, 163–177, doi:10.1016/j.schres.2007.09.031 (2008).

696 Woodley, M. A., Rindermann, H., Bell, E., Stratford, J. & Piffer, D. The relationship between microcephalin, ASPM and intelligence: a reconsideration. *Intelligence* **44**, 51–63, doi:10.1016/j.intell.2014.02.011 (2014).

697 Kanazawa, S. Intelligence and childlessness. *Social Science Research* **48**, 157–170, doi:dx.doi.org/10.1016/j.ssresearch.2014.06.003 (2014).

698 Ramsden, S. *et al.* The influence of reading ability on subsequent changes in verbal IQ in the teenage years. *Developmental Cognitive Neuroscience* **6**, 30–39, doi:10.1016/j.dcn.2013.06.001 (2013).

699 Jaeggi, S. M., Buschkuehl, M., Jonides, J. & Perrig, W. J. Improving fluid intelligence with training on working memory. *Proc. Natl. Acad. Sci. U.S.A.* **105**, 6829–6833 (2008).

700 Jaeggi, S. M., Buschkuehl, M., Jonides, J. & Shah, P. Short- and long-term benefits of cognitive training. *Proc. Natl. Acad. Sci. U.S.A.* **108**, 10081–10086, doi:10.1073/pnas.1103228108 (2011).

701 Woodley, M. A. A life history model of the Lynn-Flynn effect. *Personality and Individual Differences* **53**, 152–156, doi:10.1016/j.paid.2011.03.028 (2012).

702 Pietschnig, J. & Gittler, G. A reversal of the Flynn effect for spatial perception in German-speaking countries: evidence from a cross-temporal IRT-based meta-analysis (1977–2014). *Intelligence* **53**, 145–153, doi:10.1016/j.intell.2015.10.004 (2015).

703 Kundakovic, M. & Champagne, F. A. Early-life experience, epigenetics, and the developing brain. *Neuropsychopharmacology* **40**, 141–153, doi:10.1038/npp.2014.140 (2015).

704 Franklin, T. B. *et al.* Epigenetic transmission of the impact of early stress across generations. *Biological Psychiatry* **68**, 408–415, doi:10.1016/j.biopsych.2010.05.036 (2010).

705 Cowan, C. S. M., Callaghan, B. L., Kan, J. M. & Richardson, R. The lasting impact of early-life adversity on individuals and their descendants: potential mechanisms and hope for intervention. *Genes Brain and Behavior* **15**, 155–168, doi:10.1111/gbb.12263 (2016).

706 Yehuda, R. *et al.* Influences of maternal and paternal PTSD on epigenetic regulation of the glucocorticoid receptor gene in holocaust survivor offspring. *Am. J. Psychiat.* **171**, 872–880, doi:10.1176/appi.ajp.2014.13121571 (2014).

707 Gershon, N. B. & High, P. C. Epigenetics and child abuse: modern-day Darwinism: the miraculous ability of the human genome to adapt, and then adapt again. *American Journal of Medical Genetics Part C-Seminars in Medical Genetics* **169**, 353–360, doi:10.1002/ajmg.c.31467 (2015).

708 Ruden, D. M. The (new) new synthesis and epigenetic capacitors of morphological evolution. *Nature genetics* **43**, 88–89, doi:10.1038/ng0211-88 (2011).

709 Smith, M. E. & Farah, M. J. Are prescription stimulants "smart pills"? The epidemiology and cognitive neuroscience of prescription stimulant use by normal healthy individuals. *Psychological Bulletin* **137**, 717–741, doi:10.1037/a0023825 (2011).

710 Fox, D. Neuroscience brain buzz. *Nature* **472**, 156–158 (2011).

711 Utz, K. S., Dimova, V., Oppenlander, K. & Kerkhoff, G. Electrified minds: transcranial direct current stimulation (tDCS) and Galvanic Vestibular Stimulation (GVS) as methods of non-invasive brain stimulation in neuropsychology: A review of current data and future implications. *Neuropsychologia* **48**, 2789–2810, doi:10.1016/j.neuropsychologia.2010.06.002 (2010).

712 Clark, V. P. *et al.* TDCS guided using fMRI significantly accelerates learning to identify concealed objects. *Neuroimage* **59**, 117–128, doi:dx.doi.org/10.1016/j.neuroimage.2010.11.036 (2012).

713 Chi, R. P. & Snyder, A. W. Facilitate insight by non-invasive brain stimulation. *PLOS ONE* **6**, doi:e16655 10.1371/journal.pone.0016655 (2011).

714 Cohen Kadosh, R., Soskic, S., Iuculano, T., Kanai, R. & Walsh, V. Modulating neuronal activity produces specific and long-lasting changes in numerical competence. *Curr. Biol.* **20**, 2016–2020, doi:dx.doi.org/10.1016/j.cub.2010.10.007 (2010).

715 Iuculano, T. & Cohen Kadosh, R. The mental cost of cognitive enhancement. *The Journal of Neuroscience* **33**, 4482–4486, doi:10.1523/jneurosci.4927–12.2013 (2013).

716 Heinrichs, J. H. The promises and perils of non-invasive brain stimulation. *Int. J. Law Psychiatr.* **35**, 121–129, doi:10.1016/j.ijlp.2011.12.006 (2012).

717 Warwick, K. *et al.* Thought communication and control: a first step using radiotelegraphy. *Iee Proceedings-Communications* **151**, 185–189, doi:10.1049/ip-com.20040409 (2004).

718 Liang, P. *et al.* CRISPR/Cas9-mediated gene editing in human tripronuclear zygotes. *Protein & Cell* **6**, 363–372, doi:10.1007/s13238-015-0153-5 (2015).

719 Lanphier, E., Urnov, F., Ehlen Haecker, S. E., Werner, M. & Smolenski, J. Comment: don't edit the human germ line. *Nature* **519**, 410–411 (2015).

720 Martikainen, M. & Pedersen, O. Germline edits: heat does not help debate. *Nature* **520**, 623 (2015).

721 Cyranoski, D. & Reardon, S. Chinese scientists genetically modify human embryos. (2015). www.nature.com/news/chinese-scientists-genetically-modify-human-embryos-1.17378.

722 Harris, J. Germline manipulation and our future worlds. *Am. J. Bioeth.* **15**, 30–34, doi:10.1080/15265161.2015.1104163 (2015). [Quoted material can be found on pp. 31 and 33.]

723 Card, D. E. in *The handbook of labor economics*, Vol. 3a (eds O. Ashenfelter & D. E. Card) (Elsevier/North Holland, 1999).

724 Brown, S. R. The influence of homebuyer education on default and foreclosure risk: a natural experiment. *J. Policy Anal. Manage.* **35**, 145–172, doi:10.1002/pam.21877 (2016).

725 WHO. *Closing the gap in a generation: Health equity through action on the social determinants of health (Final Report)* (World Health Organisation, 2008).

726 Gakidou, E., Cowling, K., Lozano, R. & Murray, C. J. L. Increased educational attainment and its effect on child mortality in 175 countries between 1970 and 2009: a systematic analysis. *Lancet* **376**, 959–974, doi:10.1016/s0140-6736(10)61257-3 (2010).

727 OECD. *Improving health and social cohesion through education* (Organisation for Economic Co-operation and Development, 2010).

728 Cutler, D. M. & Lleras-Muney, A. *Education and health: Insights from international comparisons* (National Bureau of Economic Research, 2012).

729 Cleland, J. G. & Vanginneken, J. K. Maternal education and child survival in developing countries: the search for pathways of influence. *Social Science & Medicine* **27**, 1357–1368, doi:10.1016/0277-9536(88)90201-8 (1988).

730 Meyer, A. Does education increase pro-environmental behavior? Evidence from Europe. *Ecol. Econ.* **116**, 108–121, doi:10.1016/j.ecolecon.2015.04.018 (2015).

731 Stringer, M. *et al.* Parental and school effects on children's political attitudes in Northern Ireland. *British Journal of Educational Psychology* **80**, 223–240, doi:10.1348/000709909x477233 (2010).

732 Cunha, F., Heckman, J. J. & Schennach, S. M. Estimating the technology of cognitive and noncognitive skill formation. *Econometrica* **78**, 883–931, doi:10.3982/ecta6551 (2010).

733 McKeown, S., Stringer, M. & Cairns, E. Classroom segregation: where do students sit and how is this related to group relations? *Br. Educ. Res. J.* **42**, 40–55, doi:10.1002/berj.3200 (2016).

734 Pritchett, L. *The rebirth of education: School ain't learning* (Centre for Global Development, 2013).

INDEX

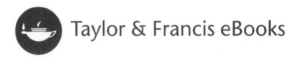

Taylor & Francis eBooks

Helping you to choose the right eBooks for your Library

Add Routledge titles to your library's digital collection today. Taylor and Francis ebooks contains over 50,000 titles in the Humanities, Social Sciences, Behavioural Sciences, Built Environment and Law.

Choose from a range of subject packages or create your own!

Benefits for you

» Free MARC records
» COUNTER-compliant usage statistics
» Flexible purchase and pricing options
» All titles DRM-free.

REQUEST YOUR FREE INSTITUTIONAL TRIAL TODAY

Free Trials Available
We offer free trials to qualifying academic, corporate and government customers.

Benefits for your user

» Off-site, anytime access via Athens or referring URL
» Print or copy pages or chapters
» Full content search
» Bookmark, highlight and annotate text
» Access to thousands of pages of quality research at the click of a button.

eCollections – Choose from over 30 subject eCollections, including:

Archaeology	Language Learning
Architecture	Law
Asian Studies	Literature
Business & Management	Media & Communication
Classical Studies	Middle East Studies
Construction	Music
Creative & Media Arts	Philosophy
Criminology & Criminal Justice	Planning
Economics	Politics
Education	Psychology & Mental Health
Energy	Religion
Engineering	Security
English Language & Linguistics	Social Work
Environment & Sustainability	Sociology
Geography	Sport
Health Studies	Theatre & Performance
History	Tourism, Hospitality & Events

For more information, pricing enquiries or to order a free trial, please contact your local sales team: www.tandfebooks.com/page/sales